NORFOLK COUNTY
WITHDRAWN FOR

The
Mother & Baby
Book of

PREGNANCY AND BIRTH

Patsy Westcott

GRAFTON BOOKS
A Division of the Collins Publishing Group

LONDON GLASGOW
TORONTO SYDNEY AUCKLAND

Grafton Books
A Division of the Collins Publishing Group
8 Grafton Street, London W1X 3LA

A Grafton Paperback Original 1990

Copyright © Argus Consumer Publications Ltd 1990

A CIP catalogue record for this book
is available from the British Library

ISBN 0-586-20661-2

Printed and bound in Great Britain by
Collins, Glasgow

Set in Goudy Old Style

All rights reserved. No part of this publication
may be reproduced, stored in a retrieval system,
or transmitted, in any form, or by any means,
electronic, mechanical, photocopying, recording or
otherwise, without the prior permission of
the publishers.

This book is sold subject to the condition that
it shall not, by way of trade or otherwise, be
lent, re-sold, hired out or otherwise circulated
without the publisher's prior consent in any
form of binding or cover other than that
in which it is published and without a similar
condition including this condition being
imposed on the subsequent purchaser.

NORFOLK LIBRARY AND INFORMATION SERVICE	
SUPPLIER	H J
INVOICE No.	229645
ORDER DATE	24.5.90
COPY No.	

Contents

Introduction	vii

Part I – PREGNANCY

How the baby grows and develops	3
The amazing placenta	7
Finding out you are pregnant	11
All about antenatal care	17
Special tests	23
Birth choices	34
Feeding	50
Looking after yourself	55
Exercise during pregnancy	67
Classes for birth preparation	74
Making the most of your appearance	77
Minor ailments of pregnancy – an A–Z	81
Miscarriage	86
The Rhesus factor	88
Worrying symptoms: what they mean	89
Preparing for your baby	92
What to buy for your baby	94
Your feelings during pregnancy	98
Your sex life	101
Rights and benefits at work	102

Part II – LABOUR AND BIRTH

Presentation	113
Twins	115
Positions for labour	117
Labour	119
The birth	138
When a baby dies	141
When labour is more complicated	142
If your baby is born too soon	152

Part III – YOU AND YOUR NEW BABY

Your new baby	157

CONTENTS

New baby check-ups	160
Establishing feeding	162
Your body	173
Back home	178
You and your husband – now that you're parents	183
Your postnatal check-up	185
Contraception	186
If the blues don't go away	188
Becoming parents	190
Glossary	195
Useful addresses	203
Useful reading	205
Index	207

Introduction

Before you become pregnant, children tend to be something other people have. Once conception occurs, however, a subtle change takes place. Suddenly a whole world which was previously invisible appears before your eyes: you notice pregnant women in the street, prams in supermarkets, toddlers playing in the park. And as you enter this new and mystifying world you didn't know existed, you become aware of how little you know about it. With today's smaller families, and the habit of children moving away from home to pursue higher education or a job, many men and women grow up having had very little to do with babies and small children, and with only the haziest idea of the sort of impact a baby will have on their lives. What's more, with the explosion of new scientific research and technology, practices change from one generation to another. Couples about to become parents need up-to-date information and support to help them cope with the changes that await them. These are what this book sets out to provide.

It is divided into three chronological parts. In the first part, dealing with pregnancy, the choices that are available in antenatal care are outlined. Decisions made at this stage can influence the sort of birth you eventually have, and it is hoped that the information given will help you evaluate the various options so that you can decide what is right for you.

This part of the book details what is going on at every stage of pregnancy and offers a wealth of advice on how to cope with both physical and emotional changes. Of course, pregnancy is not always straightforward, so there is advice to help you recognize and interpret potentially worrying symptoms and decide when to seek medical help, and information on what sort of treatment is available.

There is also plenty of practical advice on pregnancy: hints on how to look after yourself, what exercise you can take, what clothes are most practical, how to manage at work, how to find your way around the maze of maternity rights and benefits, and so on. Substantial space is devoted to helping you prepare both for the birth and for the impact your baby will have upon your life. This forms a lead into the second part of the book which deals with labour and birth. The three stages of labour are explained, and there is advice on how to recognize when you are in labour, when to take yourself to hospital, and what to expect when you get there. Pain is something that worries many women as labour approaches, and this book shows you how you and your birth companion can cope, what methods of pain relief are available, and the pros and cons of different methods. Every labour is, of course, unique, and this is recognized in the book. There are descriptions of different types of labours, and what you can expect if labour is not straightforward.

In the third part of this book the vital days and weeks after birth are covered. This is the time when you begin to get to know and love your baby. It is also a period when you may be beset by worries. Part three contains practical advice on how to organize yourself and your life to enable you to concentrate on looking after your new baby. Since feeding takes up so much time during the early weeks, plenty of information on how to make breast- or bottle-feeding a happy and enjoyable experience is included.

Of course it takes two to make a baby, and although this book is addressed primarily to women, the vital role fathers have to play is acknowledged. There is information on the changes pregnancy and birth can effect on a couple's relationship, and tips on how they can support and help each other as they journey through this new territory. Couples are referred to as husbands and wives throughout the text, simply because marriage is still the most common relationship among men and women having a child together. However, the information isn't confined to husbands and wives, and applies just as much to any other sort of partnership, or indeed to single parents.

Pregnancy is a normal process and not an illness. However, the bodily changes that take place have become 'medicalized'. Being pregnant and giving birth bring women into extensive contact with the medical profession for perhaps the first time in their lives. It can come as something of a shock to discover that what to the woman involved is an intimate, mysterious experience, is for the professional an everyday event, something to be quantified and (some would argue) reduced to observable facts and figures. Medical care has revolutionized childbirth: today relatively few babies and even fewer mothers suffer severe illness or lose their lives at this time, as happened in the past. Technology has made it possible for babies born after just 24 weeks in the womb to survive and flourish. New discoveries are helping to solve the mysteries of pre-eclampsia and recurrent miscarriage, conditions responsible for much of the toll of misery and ill-health in the past. The system of antenatal care we have in this country is second to none, yet many women complain of feeling taken over and overwhelmed. This book, which was written with the help of *Mother & Baby* magazine's medical experts, GP-obstetrician Dr Alexander Gunn and midwife and health visitor Jenny Jeffs, describes in detail the medical care you can expect, in order to help you find your way confidently around the system. Medical jargon has been kept to a minimum, but knowing the correct names for what is happening to you can help you to deal with your medical advisers as an equal partner rather than merely a passive patient. Technical terms and expressions are explained as they appear in the text. Where this would have made for clumsy or disjointed reading, page references are given. There is also a glossary where you can find brief explanations of terms used in the book and a few others that you may encounter in your dealings with medical staff.

Becoming a parent is one of the most dramatic turning points in adult life. I hope that this book will give you both the knowledge and the skill to enjoy it, and to wonder at the miracle of new life that you have created.

Patsy Westcott, 1990

Note: In order to reflect the experiences of all mothers, 'he' and 'she' have been alternated chapter by chapter in this book to refer to the baby.

Part I

PREGNANCY

How the baby grows and develops

Your baby grows more rapidly during the course of pregnancy than at any other time in his life. As well as growing in size, your baby develops from two single cells invisible to the naked eye to a fully formed human being weighing approximately 3.4 kg (7 lb. 7 oz.).

Pregnancy is dated from the first day of your last period but, in fact, conception occurs about midway through your cycle.

Two weeks Conception: a single sperm penetrates the ovum. The nucleus of the sperm merges with the nucleus of your egg to form a cell structure about 0.12 mm (1/200 in.) in size.

Three weeks Implantation: seven days after fertilization, the ball of cells (called a blastocyst), which will become your baby and the placenta, has travelled down the fallopian tube and embeds in the wall of the uterus (womb). As this happens you may lose a drop or two of blood, which you may mistake for the start of your period.

Four weeks The developing embryo is just visible to the human eye. The cells, which will later form the placenta, produce human chorionic gonadotrophin (HCG), the pregnancy hormone, and this can be detected by a urine or blood test.

Five weeks Your baby's nervous system begins to form, and a blood vessel develops that will become your baby's heart. Your baby measures just 2 mm (0.08 in.).

Six weeks Your baby is now 5 mm (0.02 in.) long. He has a head and neck, with primitive eyes and ears. His heart is already beating and its movements can be picked up on an ultrasound scan. He has a blood stream, digestive organs, liver and kidneys.

Seven weeks The baby is recognizably a human being, with organs continuing to develop. He has nostrils, lips and a tongue, and his teeth are beginning to form in his jaw. He has arms and legs, although his hands and feet are still undeveloped.

Eight weeks All your baby's major organs have formed. His eyes already have some pigment, but they are still covered by a layer of skin that will eventually become his eyelids. He is beginning to stretch his limbs and, although you are not yet aware of this development, the movements can be picked up on an ultrasound scan. He is 17 mm (0.67 in.) long. During the ensuing weeks your baby continues to grow and develop.

Twelve weeks A tiny but perfect baby has formed. From now on your baby, previously called an embryo, will be known as a fetus. His head is still big in relation to his body, and his limbs are tiny. His muscles begin to develop and grow as he moves around in the uterus. He has fingers and toes, although they are still joined by webs of skin. Your baby's sex is determined at the moment of conception, and now the genitals are formed, although it's not easy to see whether the baby is a boy or a girl. His heart is fully formed and pumps blood through his circulatory system and to and from the placenta via the umbilical cord. This will be your baby's lifeline until he is born. By the end of this week his fingers and toes will be separate digits. Your baby is 75 mm (3 in.) long and weighs just 28 g (1 oz.).

16 weeks Your baby's skin is beginning to be covered by a fine layer of downy hair called lanugo. His eyes are still closed, and his eyebrows and eyelashes are just visible. His finger- and toenails are now fully grown. He continues to move around in his bag of water (amniotic fluid) and you may be aware of a faint fluttering if this is your second or a subsequent baby. An experienced ultrasound operator may be able to tell your baby's sex by looking at a scan, although you probably won't be given the information unless you specially request it. Your baby is 15 cm (6 in.) long and weighs 114 g (4 oz.).

20 weeks Your baby weighs 227 g (8 oz.) and is 25 cm (10 in.) long. By now his movements are unmistakable. His head is about a third of the size of his whole body. He swallows amniotic fluid, and his kidneys process this to produce weak urine. The hair on his head is beginning to grow, and he may be starting to suck his thumb.

24 weeks Your baby is about 33 cm (13 in.) long and weighs about 500 g (1 lb. 2 oz.). He is covered in a thick protective layer of cream called vernix, which prevents his skin from drying out and wrinkling. His body is thin. His eyes are still closed and look rather bulging, because the chubby cheeks have not yet developed. The midwife can hear his heart through her stethoscope and may be able to determine the way in which he is lying by feeling your abdomen.

28 weeks If your baby were to be born now he would stand about a 60 per cent chance of survival, and greater in some intensive care baby units. Some babies who are born even earlier have been known to survive, given extra special care. Of course, the baby would have to spend many weeks in an incubator, which simulates the warmth and security of the womb. Your baby weighs 1000 g (2 lb. 4 oz.), and his body is now starting to grow faster than his head as it lays down fat in preparation for birth. Your baby now occupies the whole of your uterus.

32 weeks Your baby is now almost recognizably of newborn proportions. His lungs are beginning to mature, and he continues to lay down fat. He practises breathing in and out, and you may be aware of his having hiccups from time to time. He weighs 1800 g (4 lb.) and if born now he would stand a very good chance of survival, although he would still need to be nursed in a special care unit.

36 weeks By now your baby will probably have settled into position ready to be born, with his head engaged in your pelvis if he is your first baby. His lungs are almost fully mature, his kidneys are operational and his liver is beginning to deal with some of the waste produced by his body. His movements have become limited as there is now no space in the uterus for the vigorous tumbling and turning of his early months. He opens and shuts his eyes, and you may notice periods of sleeping when he becomes quiet and doesn't move.

40 weeks Your baby has reached 'term'. Most babies are born within two weeks either side of this date. He is eight times longer than he was at 12 weeks, and his weight has increased 600-fold. Most of the fine, downy hair covering his body has disappeared, although there may be traces of it on his back and shoulders. The vernix, too, is beginning to dissolve in the amniotic fluid, although patches of this creamy coating may still be present at birth.

No one knows quite what starts off labour. It's thought that it may be

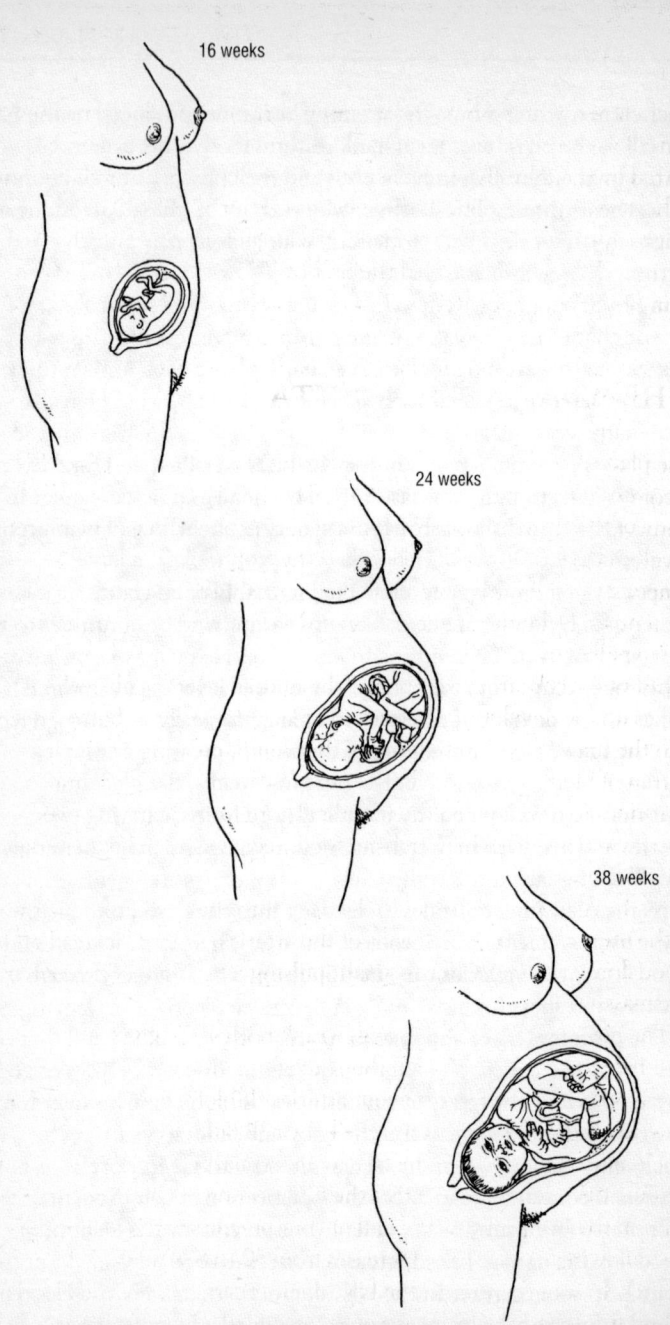

biochemical changes brought about by hormones produced by the baby himself, once he is fully developed. Alternatively, labour may be started by the ageing of the placenta and the consequent reduction in its hormone output. The average baby is about 50 cm (20 in.) long and weighs 3.4 kg (7 lb. 7 oz.) at birth. His fingernails may already need cutting when he is born, and the hair on his head may be as long as 4 cm (1½ in.).

THE AMAZING PLACENTA

The placenta is your baby's lifeline during pregnancy, and doctors are becoming increasingly convinced that the placenta holds the key to many of the things that can go wrong during pregnancy. The placenta develops from a cluster of cells called the trophoblast, a large, temporary gland, unique in biological terms. Like all glands its job is to regulate body functions but unlike other glands, once its job is finished it is expelled from the body.

Just one week after conception, the middle layer of cells, which makes up the developing embryo and placenta, starts to burrow deep into the juicy, blood-rich lining of the womb, creating a complex warren of blood vessels. Over the next few weeks, the placenta continues to develop and the umbilical cord forms, carrying two arteries and a vein, which transfer food, oxygen and waste materials to and from your baby.

As the placenta continues to dig deep into the thick, muscular wall of the uterus, it softens the walls of the arteries, so that, instead of the blood flowing to your baby in small, pulsing jets, it surges through in one massive wave.

The placenta is like a sponge in which both your blood and that of your baby is absorbed, though they never mix directly. This sponge-like lake is served by the rivers of your arteries. If blood flow is sluggish the lake may become stagnant and the baby will fail to thrive. The biochemical changes so induced can give rise to pre-eclampsia, a blood pressure disorder that can affect the functioning of your placenta.

From the beginning to the end of your pregnancy the amount of blood flowing to your baby increases from 60 to 600 ml (2½ fl. oz. to 1 pint). In some centres in the UK, doctors can measure the blood flow to and from the baby by means of a scan called a Doppler.

PREGNANCY

By the end of pregnancy your placenta measures some 15–20 cm (6–8 in.) across and is about 2.5 cm (1 in.) thick.

Functions of the placenta
- Secretes hormones that maintain the pregnancy and prevent menstruation.
- Stimulates the production of milk.
- Supplies your baby with food and oxygen and removes waste products.
- Forms a filter that prevents harmful organisms from reaching your baby. Antibodies to many of the diseases you have had pass through, giving your baby immunity in the months after birth until her own immune system takes over.

Doctors now believe that the placenta holds the secret to many problems in pregnancy, such as miscarriage, failure of the baby to grow, and the development of pre-eclampsia. In the years to come, research will bring us nearer to solving these problems.

HOW YOU CHANGE DURING PREGNANCY

Signs and symptoms	*Action*
The early weeks *Weeks 1–4* Missed period. Breasts become bigger and may tingle. Nausea and vomiting. Tiredness.	Carry out a home pregnancy test and/or make an appointment to see your doctor. See tips on page 84. Take extra rest.
Week 8 Nausea and vomiting. Urinary frequency. Breasts continue to enlarge.	Continue to follow tips on page 84. Buy yourself a larger bra.
Week 12 Nausea and vomiting may stop.	Go for booking visit to hospital.

HOW YOU CHANGE DURING PREGNANCY

Your uterus starts to rise above your pubic bone.

Your nipples become larger and darker. Small raised bumps appear in the area around the nipple. Other areas of pigment may appear on your face and abdomen, especially if you are dark-haired.

Loosen waistbands and consider buying maternity clothes. See page 53.

Middle pregnancy

Weeks 13–16
Morning sickness should begin to ease. You should start feeling more energetic as early tiredness passes. Your breasts and your uterus continue to enlarge.

You may feel more like exercising now (see tips on page 69). There may be an early pregnancy class you can attend in your area. Ask the midwife, or if you are attending active or natural birth classes (see page 74), contact the relevant organization. By now you will need to start adapting your clothes or to buy special maternity outfits.

Weeks 16–20
You may find you sweat more than usual due to the increased activity of sweat glands during pregnancy. You may suffer from some of the minor discomforts of pregnancy, such as stuffy nose, indigestion, and so on. You'll probably feel fit and well otherwise. As your baby grows and your abdomen expands your navel gradually flattens. It will return to normal once you have had your baby.

Shower daily and wear loose clothes in natural fibres. You'll probably have a scan at the 16-week antenatal check. You may be able to have a photograph of your baby taken on this occasion (some hospitals ask for payment of a small fee to offset costs).

Start setting aside time for regular relaxation. Book antenatal classes if you haven't already done so. Clean your navel gently with a piece of cotton wool moistened with warm water.

Weeks 20–24
As the baby takes up more space in your abdomen, heartburn may become a problem. Towards the end of this period the doctor or

See page 83 for tips on dealing with heartburn. If these don't help, your doctor may suggest a mild antacid.

PREGNANCY

midwife will be able to hear your baby's heart through a fetal stethoscope. Your uterus has now risen just above your navel.

Continue attending antenatal appointments. Make a note of any questions you want to ask.

The last three months

Weeks 24–28
Cramp may become a problem, and there may be a return of urinary frequency.

You'll be growing steadily bigger and putting on weight at about 500 g (1 lb.) a week.
Colostrum, the pre-milk fluid, may leak and form crusts on your nipples.

Avoid stretching your toes downwards and see page 82 for other tips.
Visit the lavatory regularly to minimize the chance of developing a urine infection.
Go shopping for your baby's layette before you get too big.

Wash nipples with plain water only and gently remove crusts. You can apply a lanolin-based cream if you wish.
Apply now for maternity benefits (see page 102). You'll probably leave work at about the 28th week. Rest and relax, but plan a few light activities so you don't get bored.

Weeks 28–32
You feel more uncomfortable as the baby puts pressure on your internal organs.

You become aware of your uterus tightening at intervals, especially when you sit or lie down. These contractions, which help prepare your uterus for labour, are known as Braxton-Hicks.
Your baby is very active. As the growing uterus pushes up against your diaphragm and ribs, you may feel breathless, especially when you climb stairs, or exert yourself. This will pass off when the baby's head becomes engaged and you will feel more comfortable.

Try to stand upright to avoid emphasizing the hollow in your back, which may cause backache. Wear low-heeled shoes.
Use these to practise relaxing during a contraction.

If you are having problems sleeping because of your baby's activity and the discomfort of your bump, wind down slowly and have a milky drink or herbal tea such as camomile prior to going to bed.
Start attending antenatal classes if you have not already done so.

Weeks 33–36
As your baby's space becomes tighter you may see hands and feet appearing as bumps on your abdomen as the baby moves around. Backache may be a problem due to the general softening of your joints.

Towards the end of this period, if this is your first baby, the head may engage in position, ready for birth, and you will feel more comfortable.

Continue attending antenatal appointments and classes. When the course ends make a note of some of the other students' names and addresses so you can stay in touch after your babies are born. Find out about local toddler clubs, postnatal support groups and so on, now before you get too tired. They are an invaluable lifeline after your baby's birth.

Watch your posture. Get your husband to massage your back if backache is troublesome.

Weeks 37–40
Your baby starts to move less as space becomes even more restricted. You may feel a strange, grinding sensation low in your pelvis as the baby moves her head low down in your uterus. Braxton-Hicks contractions become longer and stronger, and one day soon may meld into the true contractions of labour. You feel big and tired, and you can't wait for your baby to be born. On the other hand, you feel you're not really ready!

Pack your case and make final preparations for your baby's arrival. Arrange for your other children to be taken care of when you go into hospital. Continue rest and relaxation as before. Plan a few activities around the time of your baby's expected arrival date, to prevent boredom and impatience from setting in.

FINDING OUT YOU ARE PREGNANT

If you've been trying for a baby you've probably been waiting with bated breath every month to see if your period arrives. On the other hand, pregnancy may have taken you by surprise, and the failure of your period to turn up on time, followed by other signs, may have led you to suspect that you may be pregnant.

Whether your pregnancy was planned or an accident, the sooner you find out for sure the sooner you'll be able to start taking care of yourself and your unborn baby. During the first few weeks of pregnancy, your baby grows from a tiny dot, invisible to the naked eye, to a small but recognizable human being. It's during these first 12 weeks that the baby's limbs, head, brain and all other major organs are formed. After that, all he has to do is grow until he is mature enough to be born. So it's specially important that you lead a healthy life during this time and don't do anything that could adversely affect your baby's development.

Testing for pregnancy

The doctor won't usually be able to confirm your pregnancy by a physical examination alone before you are at least 6–10 weeks pregnant. However, with the methods of testing a sample of urine that are now available, there's no need to wait and wonder.

You can buy a variety of home pregnancy-testing kits from the chemist. Most kits contain two tests, so that if the first one proves negative you can try again a couple of weeks later.

The most sensitive of these tests can show whether you are pregnant as early as the day after your period was due. Some tests use a simple colour change to let you know whether you are pregnant, and they are extremely simple to carry out. Others work by showing a brown ring in the bottom of a test tube when you have conceived. Generally you will have to wait until your period is several days overdue before you can use this type of test.

The tests work by picking up the presence of a hormone called human chorionic gonadotrophin (HCG), which is produced by the embryo during the first 10 weeks of pregnancy and excreted in your urine. The best urine for the test is the first urine of the day, which is the most concentrated.

You can also have a test carried out at a chemist, at your local family planning clinic or by your GP once your period is a week or so overdue. In most areas this service is free, although pressures on hospital laboratories may mean you have to wait one or two days for the result.

SYMPTOMS OF EARLY PREGNANCY

Without the confirmation of a special test, there are several bodily changes that are clues to pregnancy. They are:

Lack of period

For most women this is the first sign, although some mothers-to-be claim to know instinctively from the moment they conceive. During the first couple of months of pregnancy, some women experience a little 'breakthrough bleeding' at about the time their period would have been due. Such bleeding is generally lighter and shorter than a proper period, but it can cause confusion over dates. However, any confusion can be cleared up by an ultrasound scan (see page 26) when you visit the antenatal clinic.

You may also notice that the pre-menstrual symptoms you normally experience, such as heavy breasts, a bloated feeling, and so on, are more pronounced than usual – and don't pass off in the usual way.

Breast changes

The hormones circulating around your system cause your breasts to start increasing the size of secretory glandular tissue and laying down extra milk-producing cells in preparation for feeding your baby. Your breasts will feel tight, full and uncomfortable, and you will see veins beneath the skin caused by the increased blood flow to them. By the time your second or third period would have been due, you will probably need to wear a larger bra.

You'll also notice that your nipples are more prominent and that the ring surrounding them, the areola, is darker in colour than usual. This may be specially noticeable if you are dark-haired or dark-skinned.

If you look carefully you can see small, raised bumps around the nipple. These are special skin glands that, later on in pregnancy, secrete a lubricating substance designed to keep your nipples soft and supple for breast-feeding.

Nausea and vomiting

You may feel queasy or even be sick. In fact, 'morning sickness', which affects about half of all mothers-to-be, often doesn't occur in the mornings at all but throughout the day or while travelling. It may be sparked off by strong smells or foods such as coffee, garlic, curry or fried foods. Tips for coping with nausea and vomiting are given on page 84.

Fatigue

During the first three months of pregnancy you may feel totally exhausted. Even the simplest things seem an effort. However, it's hardly surprising, for during this time your baby is growing more rapidly than he will ever again in his life, and drawing on your energy reserves in the process. The hormone balance of your body is changing dramatically, and it also takes a little while to become emotionally adjusted to the idea that you are expecting a baby.

Urinary frequency

You may suddenly find yourself needing to empty your bladder far more frequently than usual. The symptom is caused by pressure on your bladder from your uterus as it becomes enlarged. It is also in part due to an increase in blood flow to the bladder, caused by circulation changes.

CONFIRMATION OF PREGNANCY

When your period is two weeks overdue or as soon as you suspect you are pregnant, you should make an appointment to see your GP. He or she will be the link between you and the hospital specialists and will be a great source of support and advice during your pregnancy and after the birth of your baby. He or she will be able to link you into the formal system of antenatal care and help you to decide how this should be organized to suit your particular needs.

In most group medical practices there is at least one doctor who is specially trained in caring for pregnant women. If your pregnancy is straightforward this doctor and the practice midwife will probably undertake most of your antenatal care, although you will have to make a few visits to the hospital for special tests and detailed investigations to ensure that all is progressing as it should. This system is called shared care.

Alternatively, if there are any midwife-run clinics in your area you may attend one of these and have occasional check-ups by the GP or at the hospital.

If you have any existing health problems, or if the pregnancy is complicated in any way, all your antenatal care will probably take place at the hospital antenatal clinic, where there are experts on hand to give advice should anything go wrong. This is known as consultant care.

You'll find more details on the various types of antenatal care on page 21.

What will the doctor need to know?

Your doctor may hold a special antenatal session, or you may be asked to attend during surgery hours. At the first appointment the doctor will want to ask you a number of questions and examine you.

Wear clothes that are easy to get on and off, and take along a small sample of the first urine you pass in the morning, in a small clean container, such as an empty aspirin bottle.

Your doctor will want to know the date of the first day of your last period, in order to work out approximately when your baby is due (your Expected Date of Delivery or EDD). He or she will ask you about any signs and symptoms that you have had, and will also want to examine you to see whether your uterus is enlarged.

If you are not certain you are pregnant your GP may carry out a pregnancy test, but is more likely to send a sample of your urine to the laboratory to be tested or ask you to take a sample along yourself.

He or she will want to know a few details about your personal medical history, as well as your general well-being so far.

Your doctor will ask whether you have any preferences for the type of birth you will have, so you will need to think about this and perhaps discuss it with your husband before you make your visit. You'll find the various options described on page 34, to help you make up your mind.

Once your pregnancy has been confirmed, the doctor will write to one of the consultants at the local hospital maternity unit to make arrangements for a full assessment of your state of health and the pregnancy. This is called the booking appointment. If you are having a hospital birth arrangements will also be made for a bed to be booked for you.

When is the baby due?

Perhaps the most exciting part of the first visit is the moment your doctor tells you when you can expect your baby. Pregnancy lasts approximately 280 days, and this is measured from the first day of your last period, although conception takes place about midway between your periods.

You can calculate the date your baby is due from the chart below. Alternatively, you can do this sum:

	Example
First day of last period	1.4.1989
Plus 9 months	1.1.1990
Plus 7 days	8.1.1990

PREGNANCY

If your menstrual cycle is longer or shorter than the standard 28 days add or subtract the appropriate number of days:

	Example
35-day cycle (i.e. 7 days longer than conventional cycle)	
First day of last period	1.4.1989
Plus 9 months	1.1.1990
Plus 14 days	15.1.1990

21-day cycle (i.e. 7 days shorter than conventional cycle)
First day of last period — 1.4.1989
Plus 9 months — 1.1.1990
(There's no need to add extra days since the cycle is 7 days shorter than usual)

Do bear in mind that your expected date of delivery (EDD) is only approximate. Only a mere 5 per cent of babies are born on their precise EDD; the rest are born within a couple of weeks before or after the expected date. Some babies, of course, are premature, and a few are born more than a fortnight after the EDD and are still perfectly healthy.

At around 16 weeks of pregnancy you'll probably be given a scan, which, at this stage, will date your pregnancy extremely accurately.

Signs and symptoms of pregnancy

Tick any that you experience

- Missed period
- Sickness
- Breast changes
- Changes in taste and smell
- Tiredness
- Wanting to pass urine frequently
- Any others (make a note here of any other signs you've noticed)

....

....

....

All about antenatal care

Antenatal care is designed to give you the best possible chance of staying fit and well during pregnancy, and of giving birth to a strong and healthy baby. It's important to take full advantage of this system of medical care, which ensures that any potential problems can be spotted before they become troublesome.

Some aspects of the antenatal care system have come in for adverse criticism in recent years. Complaints of the 'production-line' atmosphere of clinics, of the lack of continuity in care and of a feeling of impersonality have led to the introduction of several welcome changes in the organization and running of many clinics.

Some hospitals are experimenting with a system of team midwifery, whereby you are looked after by the same group of midwives during pregnancy, labour and on the postnatal ward. Others run midwife-only clinics for mothers-to-be with straightforward pregnancies. In some areas, hospital consultants with their own team of midwives visit outlying surgeries and health centres, so that those women who run a high risk of developing complications have the facility of a greater degree of personal care. In other districts, women can telephone the hospital clinic with their medical readings, such as blood pressure, and so avoid having to make the journey to attend. Such changes, which are slowly taking place, should help to provide a pattern of antenatal care that meets women's individual personal as well as physical needs during pregnancy.

How often will I visit the antenatal clinic?

The normal pattern of antenatal visits is to attend for a simple check-up, as described below, once a month until you are 28 weeks pregnant. After that, you attend once a fortnight until the 36th week and, thereafter, once a week until your baby is born. Some hospitals are cutting the number of visits made by low-risk women. You may have to make one or two extra visits, to undergo any special tests that may be necessary.

What happens during an antenatal check?

At each antenatal visit the following checks are performed:

- You are weighed to check that your baby is growing normally.
- Your blood pressure is taken. This is to check for a condition called

pre-eclampsia (also known as toxaemia, a blood pressure disorder), which could lessen the blood supply to your baby.
- Your urine is tested for glucose, to ensure that you are not developing a type of pregnancy diabetes. It is also tested for the presence of proteins (albumin), which could be an indication that pre-eclampsia is developing, and to make sure there is no urine infection.
- The doctor or midwife feels your abdomen to check on the baby's size and position, and listens to her heart beat using a special stethoscope.

It's easy to forget questions in the hustle and bustle of the antenatal clinic, so make a point of listing any queries you have before you attend. Most doctors and midwives are happy to explain what is happening if you ask.

The booking visit

Your first visit to the hospital antenatal clinic takes place some time between the 12th and 16th week of pregnancy. It's intended to check on your general level of health, as this can affect the course of your pregnancy, and to make a thorough assessment of your pregnancy, to determine whether you are likely to develop any complications. You'll see a consultant obstetrician, who will examine you. You'll also probably have an ultrasound scan and various routine blood tests.

Many hospitals hold special booking-only clinics, although at some, mothers-to-be attending for repeat visits are also included. You may find that you spend a couple of hours at the clinic. Bear with this, however, as it's essential for your own and your baby's health and well-being that you have a thorough check-up at this stage.

Some clinics have videos, magazines, and a crèche for any other children you may have. However, you can't count on it. Take along a book or magazine to read, to while away the time, or go along with a friend. In many hospitals it's acceptable to take your husband to the booking clinic, and this will enable him to feel more involved with your pregnancy, as well as being company for you. If there are no child-care facilities try to get your children looked after while you visit the clinic. If you have to take them with you, pack a few books and toys, a drink and a snack to help distract them while you are being examined.

Providing personal details

The first step is to provide your personal details for your medical records. This involves spending about 20 minutes with a midwife answering questions about your previous and family medical history, and also that of your husband. Be prepared to provide the following information:

- Name, age, address, telephone number, date of birth, place of birth and job.
- The same details about your husband. (Don't forget to ask him where he was born if you don't already know.)
- Date of your marriage.
- Whether you have ever suffered any serious illnesses or accidents.
- Whether you smoke or drink and how much.
- Whether you are taking any medicines, either prescribed or over-the-counter.
- Whether there are any illnesses, such as TB, diabetes or mental illness, in your own or husband's families. (Ask your parents or parents-in-law if you're uncertain.)
- The length of your menstrual cycle and of your periods.
- Whether the pregnancy was planned.
- The date of your last period.
- The type of contraception you were using before becoming pregnant.
- Details of any previous pregnancies, miscarriages or terminations.
- How you plan to feed your baby (see page 50, to help you decide).
- How long you would like to stay in hospital, though there won't always be any choice.

You'll have the chance to ask questions, and you will be given several free leaflets about pregnancy and birth, your rights at work, and so on. The midwife may also give you some tips and advice on how to look after yourself in terms of diet and exercise.

Examinations and tests

After this, you'll have a complete physical examination. This includes:

- A blood test, to determine your blood group and red blood cell count and check for anaemia, German measles (rubella) and for syphilis or other abnormalities in your health.
- A urine test, to check for any abnormalities, as described above.

- A blood pressure check, as above.
- A check on your heart and breathing, to ensure you are in good physical health.
- An internal examination, to check that your reproductive organs are healthy and that the uterus and baby are growing as they should.
- A cervical smear test, if you haven't had one done lately.
- A check on weight and measurements, to assess the capacity of your pelvis and determine if you are likely to have a normal delivery.
- An examination of your legs, to see whether you have any varicose veins, which could become worse during pregnancy.
- An examination of your breasts, to check for any problems that may make breast-feeding difficult.
- An ultrasound scan, to assess the size of your baby and her age. This isn't always done at the booking visit. The most reliable time for predicting the baby's age is at around 16 weeks, so you may be asked to make another visit at that time (see page 26).

Arranging further visits

Finally, you'll be asked whether you plan to attend the hospital for your antenatal care, or whether you are having shared care between your family doctor and the hospital (see page 21). You'll be given a date for your next clinic visit, and if you are having shared care, a co-operation card (see pages 26–7) with brief details of the findings of this visit, which is filled in every time you go for an antenatal check.

Coping with an internal examination

An internal examination is usually carried out at your first visit to the doctor when you are 6–10 weeks pregnant. It enables the doctor accurately to assess your pregnancy and the health of your internal organs. You'll also have an internal when you go for your booking visit at the hospital antenatal clinic.

Your doctor inserts two fingers into your vagina and, at the same time, presses your abdomen with the other hand. This enables him or her to assess the size of your uterus and to detect the softness of your vagina and cervix (neck of your womb) that occurs during pregnancy.

This cannot harm the baby or you, but it's understandable if you feel a little nervous. Relax and breathe evenly in and out.

With the increased use of ultrasound scans, doctors now perform far fewer internal examinations. You may have only one or two during your entire pregnancy.

ALL ABOUT ANTENATAL CARE

Choices in antenatal care

The sort of antenatal care you are given will depend on whether your pregnancy is straightforward, or whether any medical problems are anticipated. If your pregnancy is unproblematic you may be asked to choose what sort of care you would prefer. There are advantages and disadvantages to each type of care, so you need to think carefully about which would suit you best. Take into account the distance you will have to travel. You stand a greater chance of continuity of care if you opt for shared care or midwife care.

SHARED CARE Your GP and midwife provide most of your antenatal care. The precise proportion depends to some extent on where you live and the course of your pregnancy. A typical arrangement would be to see your own doctor once a month until the 36th week and then, if you are having a hospital birth, to attend the hospital clinic weekly until the birth. You will attend hospital for your booking visit and perhaps for an additional check at 32 weeks, as well as for any special tests that may be necessary.

CONSULTANT CARE Usually this is provided only if you are having a problematical pregnancy or it is anticipated that you will have a difficult pregnancy. You may not always see the consultant – you could see one of the other doctors instead, but the consultant has overall responsibility for your care.

MIDWIFE CARE This type of antenatal care is provided at a midwife-run clinic at the hospital, at your doctor's surgery or, in some areas, at a local authority clinic. A doctor is available for back-up if any problems should arise. Your booking visit and any special tests you may need will usually take place at the hospital antenatal clinic. If you find it difficult to get to a clinic a district (community) midwife will sometimes visit you at home.

WHO'S WHO AT THE ANTENATAL CLINIC

Staff at the antenatal clinic fall into two principal categories:

- Nursing staff – mainly midwives with varying degrees of experience.
- Medical staff – doctors with varying degrees of expertise and experience.

There may also be:

- Ancillary staff.
- Specialists such as radiographers, who deal with ultrasound.
- Technicians, who take blood tests.

Nursing staff

The midwife is generally a nurse who has done the 18-month midwifery training. Some midwives go direct into midwifery, in which case training lasts three years. The midwife is an expert in normal pregnancy and childbirth and is the backbone of the antenatal clinic.

The senior midwife, who has had many years' experience, is **sister-in-charge** of the antenatal clinic and is responsible for its smooth running.

Staff midwives are fully trained midwives who take care of the practical, physical and emotional aspects of your pregnancy, and advise and help with any problems you may have.

Student midwives are nurses who are training. You may be able to tell by the number of stripes on their hats at which point they are in their training (first, second or third six-monthly period).

Student nurses also have to spend a period observing in the maternity unit.

It's easier to decipher who is who if they are wearing name badges. Most hospitals use some form of colour coding to indicate status. In some hospitals this may be a different-coloured belt worn by different grades of staff. In others the colour of the uniform is used to distinguish seniority. If you are unsure who's who, don't be afraid to ask.

Medical staff

The consultant obstetrician is at the top of the medical tree. Depending on the size of the hospital, there will be about two to five of these. Generally, each one is in charge of a ward or floor in the maternity unit. The consultant is a senior doctor with at least ten years' experience in obstetrics (care of the pregnant woman and her child). He or she is also a gynaecologist – a specialist in diseases and disorders of the female reproductive organs. The team of doctors and midwives that will care for you during your pregnancy and afterwards is led by the consultant, who is responsible for all major decisions about your medical care during pregnancy. Any special procedures that other members of the team decide you need will be referred to him or her. On your first visit to the antenatal clinic the consultant will give you a complete medical check-up, and will perform an internal examination to ensure that your pregnancy is normal. So long as your pregnancy is straightforward you can expect to see the consultant only on this

ALL ABOUT ANTENATAL CARE

occasion, and perhaps again nearer delivery. If it is anticipated that your pregnancy may have complications, or if you are a private patient, you will see the consultant at every antenatal visit.

Normally at each antenatal visit you will be seen by a registrar and/or a house officer, unless you are attending a midwives' clinic.

The registrar comes next in line to the consultant. There may be one or more of these highly qualified doctors, who are usually destined in due course to become consultants in their own right. The registrar will decide what course of action to take if you run into problems and will refer this decision to the consultant.

House officers are qualified doctors who are doing a period of training in obstetrics. They may go on to specialize, or they may become GPs or enter another speciality.

SUMMARY OF ANTENATAL TESTS

Test	What it's for	When it is done
Blood	Haemoglobin (Hb) level, to check for anaemia.	First visit and towards the end of pregnancy in normal circumstances.
	Blood group – A, B or O – and to check whether you are Rhesus negative or positive.	
	VDLR and Wassermann test, to check for syphilis.	First visit.
	Rubella, to check your immunity to German measles, which could harm your developing baby if you are in contact with it during early pregnancy and have not previously had it or been immunized against it.	First visit.
	Alpha-feto protein (AFP), to test for spina bifida, and Down's syndrome (see page 32).	16 weeks.
Blood pressure	To check for any sudden rise that might indicate the development of pre-eclampsia. Normal blood pressure is between 90/50 and 130/80.	Every visit.

SUMMARY OF ANTENATAL TESTS

Test	What it's for	When it is done
Urine	To test for protein in the urine, which could be an indication that you are developing pre-eclampsia (see page 90) or have a urine infection. To test for glucose and ketones, both of which are signs that you could be developing pregnancy diabetes (see page 92).	Every visit.
Weight	To make sure your baby is growing correctly. To pick up any sudden changes in weight that could indicate problems. A sudden increase in weight can be a sign of pre-eclampsia. Weight loss can indicate the placenta is not working as well as it should.	Every visit.
Abdominal examination	To check the size of your baby and the position in which she is lying.	Every visit.
Vaginal examination (internal)	To confirm you are pregnant. To check for normal changes in your pelvic organs. To check for any abnormalities in your reproductive organs that could cause difficulties during birth. To carry out a cervical smear and swab to detect any changes that need attention, or any infections that need to be cleared up. To check that your birth outlet is wide enough for your baby.	First visit and usually again towards the end of pregnancy.

Test	What it's for	When it is done
Ultrasound	To check your dates (baseline scan). To check that your baby is healthy and has no obvious abnormalities. To check the amount of amniotic fluid around your baby. To check your baby's size. To check your baby's position before amniocentesis (see page 29), or in later pregnancy for birth.	First visit or between about 16 and 20 weeks (baseline scan). Thereafter as necessary.
Baby's heart beat	To make sure your baby is alive and well, and that her heart rate is normal. Any change in her heart rate could indicate that she is not thriving and needs to be born as soon as possible.	Every visit.
Ankles and wrists	To check for any swelling that could be a sign of pre-eclampsia.	Every visit.
Height (and sometimes shoe size)	To give some idea of the size of your pelvis.	First visit.
Breasts	To check that your nipples and breasts are suitable for breast-feeding. If your nipples turn inwards (inverted) this can often be put right during pregnancy.	First visit.
Heart and lungs	To check your general health and for any breathing difficulties that might be a problem in labour.	First visit, at three months, six months and towards the end of pregnancy.

PREGNANCY

SPECIAL TESTS

As well as the routine tests already described, there are a number of special tests that may be carried out to check that your baby is fit and well.

ULTRASOUND SCAN

A scanner works by bouncing sound waves off a solid object to produce a picture of the inside of the body. It has been used in pregnancy for 25 years and there is no evidence that any harm has ever come to mother or baby.

Your scan may be carried out by a radiographer, or a midwife who has been specially trained to interpret scans. Alternatively, it may be done by your obstetrician.

Your co-operation card

The co-operation card contains details noted at your booking visit and further information is entered on it every time you have an antenatal check. The following are some of the abbreviations you may see on your card.

LMP	Last menstrual period.
Hb	Haemoglobin (red blood cell level).
Fe	Iron. You may see this if you have been prescribed iron tablets.
NAD	Nothing abnormal detected. Everything is straightforward and there is no sugar or protein in your urine.
EDD/EDC	Expected date of delivery or confinement.
NP	Not palpable, i.e. the baby cannot yet be felt when the midwife feels your abdomen.
FHH	Fetal heart heard.
FHNH	Fetal heart not heard. If you see this don't worry. It could be that it's too early or that your baby is lying in such a way that the heart beat is undetectable.
FMF	Fetal movement felt.
FMNF	Fetal movement not felt – again, this is nothing to worry about.
Vx/Ceph	Vertex/cephalic, i.e. your baby is positioned head down.
E/Eng	Engaged, i.e. the baby's head has descended into the pelvis ready for birth.
F/Ne	Free/Not engaged.

A baseline scan is usually done at about 16 to 20 weeks of pregnancy. At this stage it is possible to measure the age of your baby extremely accurately, in order to predict the expected date of delivery. The scan also shows whether you are expecting twins (or more), the position in which the baby is lying, and where the placenta is placed. It is essential to have information on the position of the placenta, for if it is obstructing the entrance to the womb, the baby will need to be born by caesarean (see page 148).

A scan can also be used to detect a number of abnormalities, such as spina bifida, and it can be used to guide doctors when doing an amniocentesis or chorion villus sampling (see pages 29–30).

What happens when you have a scan

You will be asked to drink about a litre (or pint and a half) of liquid, so that you have a full bladder. This is to raise the uterus above the

LOA/ROA	Left/Right occipito anterior. The back of the baby's head, the occiput, is towards the left or right of the abdomen. This is the most common position (see page 114).
LOP/ROP	Left/Right occipito posterior. The baby's back is towards your spine and she is facing towards your abdomen. This is a less common position and may result in prolonged, backache labour (see page 114).
RSA	Right sacral anterior. When your baby is lying with her bottom downwards in the breech position, her sacrum, i.e. the lower part of her back, is used to describe her position rather than her head or occiput. Right sacral anterior means the baby is lying in the breech position with her body to the right front part of your abdomen.
T	Term, i.e. 40 weeks.
Para	Parity, i.e. the number of previous pregnancies.
PP	Presenting part, i.e. the part of your baby that is lying at the bottom of the uterus.
Brim	The inlet of your pelvis.
Oedema	Swelling.
Fundus	The top of your uterus, usually measured in weeks.
BP	Blood pressure. If it exceeds 140/90 on several occasions it could be a warning sign of pre-eclampsia (toxaemia).
PET	Pre-eclamptic toxaemia, the high blood pressure disease of pregnancy (see pages 90–92).

PREGNANCY

bladder in order to pick up an image of the baby. (Ultrasound was first used by submariners to detect shoals of fish!) You then lie on a couch and the skin of your abdomen is oiled. A hand-held transducer (the arm of the scanner) is passed slowly over your abdomen and the resulting picture appears on a screen. The operator takes freeze-frame pictures or polaroids to measure the diameter of your baby's head, his girth and his length, and observes him carefully to make sure he is well. The various parts of your baby will be pointed out to you. This first view of your baby is often a very exciting and moving experience. It's usually possible to take your husband or a friend with you. Don't hesitate to ask questions.

DOPPLER ULTRASOUND

A highly specialized type of scanning has been introduced into a few top hospitals, capable of measuring the blood flow in the placenta and in the mother's and baby's veins. Over the next few years simpler versions of this equipment are likely to be available in an increasing number of maternity units and could change the face of maternity care.

Your baby's nourishment and well-being during his time in the womb is dependent on the amount of blood flowing to him via the placenta. When, at 10 to 18 weeks of pregnancy, the placenta attaches itself to the lining of the uterus and then spreads out, it softens the walls of the arteries so that instead of the blood pulsating through them in spurts, it surges through in one great wave. The Doppler scanner picks up the blood flow and can detect whether the blood vessels have opened up. If they have not opened your baby could suffer from starvation or lack of oxygen (the experts call it intrauterine growth retardation), and you are liable to suffer from high blood pressure.

A Doppler scan enables doctors to predict at an early stage (about 18

What a scan shows

- That you are pregnant.
- The age of the baby.
- The position of the baby.
- The position of the placenta.
- The number of babies you are carrying.
- Any abnormalities.
- Later on in pregnancy, the stage of development of your baby and the amount of amniotic fluid in which he is floating.

weeks) those babies who are at risk. Later on in pregnancy, the Doppler can indicate those babies who need extra help or who could benefit from early delivery.

AMNIOCENTESIS

This is a test that is advised only if you are considered to be at risk, for example if it is suspected that your baby has a chromosomal abnormality. The test can also determine the sex of your baby, so it is useful to have this information where there is a risk of sex-linked

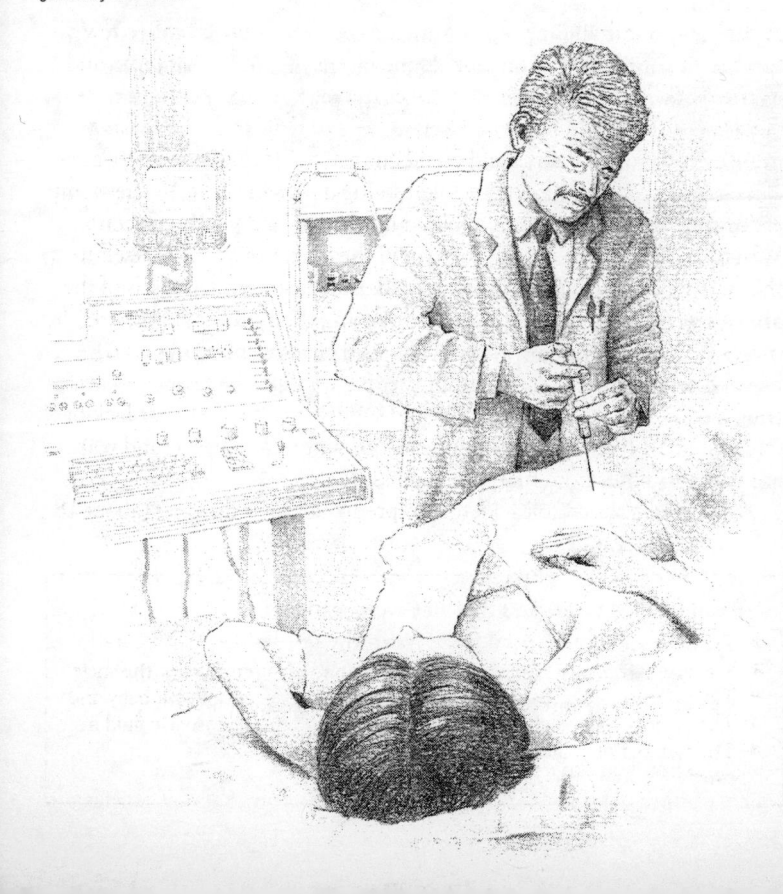

Amniocentesis. The doctor carefully removes a sample of amniotic fluid, using a needle guided by ultrasound

hereditary disorders such as haemophilia and a particular type of muscular dystrophy.

Amniocentesis is not usually carried out until the 14th to 16th week of pregnancy, though a few specialist centres are experimenting with carrying it out earlier; results take about three weeks to come through, by which time you may have already felt your baby move. For this reason, the newer chorion villus sampling (see below) is increasingly being performed to make these investigations.

The test involves passing a fine needle through the wall of the abdomen and into the uterus, and drawing off a small amount of the amniotic fluid (waters) in which your baby is floating. The surface of your skin is numbed with a local anaesthetic and the needle is carefully guided in with the aid of an ultrasound scan, to avoid puncturing the placenta.

Because of the slight danger of miscarriage – although less than one per cent – amniocentesis will probably be advised only if you have a family history of congenital abnormality, or when other tests indicate an increased risk of Down's syndrome.

If any evidence of serious abnormality is found, you'll need to consider whether or not you would have the pregnancy terminated. Counselling will be offered to help you and your husband come to a decision. If you decide on a termination you may find it hard to come to terms with the loss of your baby. You'll need plenty of support and sympathy from those around you. There is also an organization, Support After Termination For Abnormality (SAFTA), that can help you overcome the problems associated with the loss of a baby (see page 204).

CHORION VILLUS SAMPLING (CVS)

This test is becoming more widely available. It can be carried out as early as eight weeks of pregnancy, but a few centres are experimenting with doing CVS later, and this may well become more widely available; results are available in just a few days. If the results are positive and you opt for a termination at this early stage in the pregnancy, a simple suction extraction can be done under local or general anaesthetic. (This is probably less traumatic than a later termination, after 20 weeks, when you have to go through labour.)

Like amniocentesis, CVS can detect chromosomal abnormalities, such as Down's syndrome, and can also reveal the sex of your baby, which is important information if there is a history of sex-linked inherited diseases.

The test involves drawing off a small amount of the tiny, frond-like structures that anchor the baby to the wall of the uterus and later develop into the placenta. A microscopic amount of this material is gently drawn off, guided by ultrasound, either via the vagina or through a small puncture in your abdomen. It is then cultured and analysed.

The risk of miscarriage with a CVS is slightly higher than that with an amniocentesis. However, doctors consider that many of these abnormal pregnancies would naturally be terminated by miscarriage.

You will receive sympathetic counselling before the test is performed, to make sure you understand the reasons for it and the procedure, and also after the test if the results prove positive.

FETOSCOPY

This involves passing a tiny fibre-optic telescope into the uterus to observe the baby, to take blood samples, or to carry out blood transfusions on babies suffering from Rhesus disease. It is carried out at about 15 weeks. The telescope is introduced in the same way as for an amniocentesis, via the abdomen. Every part of the baby's developing brain can be observed, and a tiny drop of the baby's blood can be taken to test for blood conditions, such as thalassaemia and sickle cell disease, which affect one in ten people of Afro-Caribbean, Asian and Mediterranean origin, and brain disorders.

OESTRIOL TESTS

Oestriol is a type of oestrogen secreted by the placenta. If it is suspected that your baby is not growing properly, an oestriol level test may be carried out by taking a blood sample or collecting urine to indicate how well the placenta is functioning. However, the results of this test are not always reliable. For instance, a kidney infection can produce a low oestriol count, and drugs such as aspirin and some types of antibiotic can cause a reduction in the hormone levels too. Doctors therefore prefer to rely more on physical tests, such as ultrasound and monitoring the baby's heart beat, to check on his well-being. Alternatively, you may be asked to keep a kick chart (see page 33) to record your baby's movements. A baby who is moving vigorously is likely to be fit and well.

ALPHA-FETO PROTEIN (AFP) TEST

Alpha-feto protein is a substance produced by your developing baby that is present in your blood stream during pregnancy. A raised AFP level can indicate certain defects of the central nervous system, such as spina bifida. If the level is raised you will usually be offered an amniocentesis. A low level, combined with a low level of oestriol and high levels of the pregnancy hormone HCG can be an indication of Down's syndrome.

The test is carried out by taking a blood sample. It is usually performed at 16 weeks of pregnancy and may be repeated at intervals to check for any changes in the levels of AFP. However, the AFP levels rise as your pregnancy advances, so if you miscalculate the stage of your pregnancy you may be unnecessarily alarmed. Your AFP level will also be raised if you are expecting more than one baby.

It is therefore not a precise diagnostic test and is carried out in conjunction with other tests to confirm or refute any suspect findings.

AMNIOSCOPY

This involves examining the amniotic fluid by means of a small telescope inserted through the cervix. If the fluid contains traces of meconium it could indicate that the baby is in trouble and needs delivering immediately. Amnioscopy is a test that is only rarely carried out in the UK, although it is more common in Europe. It is carried out towards the end of pregnancy if the consultant suspects that your baby may be distressed, or if he or she is considering an induction.

STRESS TESTS

If it is suspected that your baby is overdue and is not coping well with his extra time in the womb, a drip may be set up to cause contractions. The baby's heart beat is then carefully monitored, just as it would be in labour. Under normal circumstances your baby's heart rate slows during a contraction and returns to normal when the contraction finishes. If the heart beat continues to be slow it could indicate that your baby is short of oxygen and needs to be delivered as soon as possible. In this case you will be offered an induction, or it may be decided to do an immediate caesarean section (see pages 147–50).

Kick chart

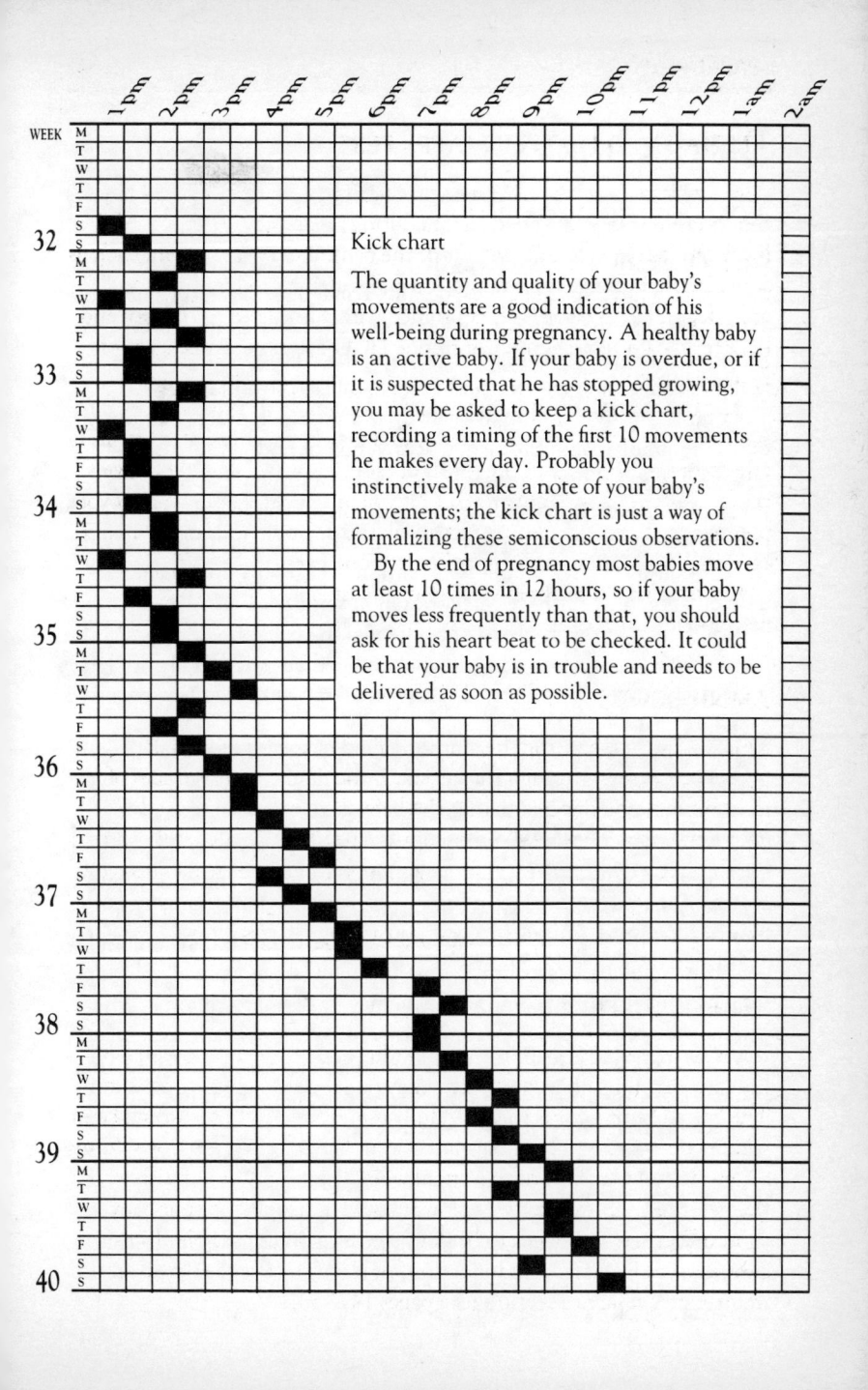

The quantity and quality of your baby's movements are a good indication of his well-being during pregnancy. A healthy baby is an active baby. If your baby is overdue, or if it is suspected that he has stopped growing, you may be asked to keep a kick chart, recording a timing of the first 10 movements he makes every day. Probably you instinctively make a note of your baby's movements; the kick chart is just a way of formalizing these semiconscious observations.

By the end of pregnancy most babies move at least 10 times in 12 hours, so if your baby moves less frequently than that, you should ask for his heart beat to be checked. It could be that your baby is in trouble and needs to be delivered as soon as possible.

Birth choices

HOME OR HOSPITAL?

One of the early decisions you will have to make is where and how you are going to have your baby. Generally, babies are born in hospital, but some mothers prefer the idea of a home birth. Some studies have shown that, provided the mother is healthy and there is no likelihood of complications, home birth can be just as safe as birth in hospital.

Complications are more likely to arise if you are having your fourth or subsequent baby, and/or if you are over 35 or under 20. However, if you are in good general health and have had a straightforward pregnancy this time, there may be no reason for you to be especially at risk. If you are expecting your first baby your body's ability to cope with the stress and strain of labour is as yet untested. Many doctors prefer to deliver women in all these categories in hospital.

You'll need to think carefully before making your choice. Discuss the matter with your doctor and midwife, and perhaps with local contacts such as a National Childbirth Trust teacher or birth group (see page 203 for addresses).

The following are the choices that are open to you.

FULL HOSPITAL CARE

This means you are booked into hospital under one of the consultants. You have your baby in hospital and receive some or all of your postnatal care there. How long you stay after the birth will depend on your and your baby's health, your choice, and how many beds are available at the time you give birth. In some areas you may be discharged home, where you will be under the care of community midwives, as little as a day after you have given birth. The maximum length of stay is 10 days, but you will only usually stay this long if you or the baby are unwell. Most women stay in for between two and five days.

HOME DELIVERY

Your antenatal care will be carried out by your GP and community midwives, who may be attached to the GP's practice. In some areas it is possible to book a private midwife, who will carry out your antenatal care and deliver you at home. You give birth at home, attended by a community midwife (often the same one whom you have met antenatally), and your GP if necessary. A community midwife will call on you twice a day for the first three days after birth, and once a day for seven days after that, to make sure that you and the baby are thriving.

DOMINO SCHEME

The Domino scheme, which stands for 'Domiciliary-in-out', operates in some areas and is a good compromise between home and hospital. Under this scheme you receive antenatal care from your local community (domiciliary) midwife, under the supervision of your GP. When you are in labour the same midwife accompanies you to the hospital or GP unit and delivers your baby. You return home between six and 48 hours later, so long as you and your baby are both well.

GP UNIT

This is a special unit, which may be part of the hospital's maternity ward, or it may be a separate unit run for the use of local GPs. Provided your pregnancy is straightforward you are looked after antenatally by your own family doctor and community midwife, who will also deliver you in the GP unit. The atmosphere is generally very free and easy, and you may be encouraged to move around and try different positions for labour. If the GP unit is part of the hospital you can easily be transferred to the consultant unit should any unexpected complications arise.

CONSULTANT UNIT

If you fall into a group with a high risk of complications, you'll be advised to have your baby in a consultant unit, where you will be under the care of one of the hospital consultants. In many hospitals, each consultant is in charge of a single ward, although the number of consultants varies depending on the size of the hospital.

PRIVATE MIDWIVES

If you can afford the cost you may like to have a home birth in the care

PREGNANCY

of a private, sometimes called an independent, midwife. A private midwife is self-employed and will provide all your antenatal and postnatal care, and will also deliver your baby.

The advantage of having a private midwife is that you will be looked after by the same person throughout your pregnancy and afterwards. You are also likely to be offered a greater choice in the way you have

---

Choosing where to have your baby

There are many considerations to take into account when deciding where you will have your baby. Top of the list are health considerations.

- Do you have a previous history of heart disease, TB, kidney disease, asthma, high blood pressure?
- Do you suffer from diabetes, epilepsy or any other chronic medical condition?
- Have you previously given birth to a stillborn baby or gone into premature labour?
- Have you previously had a difficult delivery, e.g. forceps, caesarean?
- Have you ever had a ruptured uterus or haemorrhage after birth?
- Are you Rhesus negative and your husband Rhesus positive?
- Is your baby growing as she should?
- Are you under 1.57 m (5 ft. 2 ins.), or do you take size 3 shoes or less?
- Is your baby more than a fortnight overdue?
- Are you expecting twins?
- Have you experienced any bleeding problems during this pregnancy?
- Has an ultrasound scan shown your placenta to be lying low in the uterus (placenta praevia, see page 148)?
- Have you had very high blood pressure or pre-eclampsia during this pregnancy?

If you have answered yes to any of these questions you would be well advised on medical grounds to have your baby in hospital.

When making the decision on where to have your baby, you should also take into account the following practical considerations:

- Do you have hot and cold running water in your home, preferably near the room where you would give birth?
- Do you have someone to stay with you during labour?
- How easily can you arrange for your other children to be looked after?
- Do you have someone who can help at home and look after you after the baby is born?
- How far do you live from the hospital? Is there an obstetric flying squad in your area, i.e. an ambulance and team to come to your home equipped to deal with any emergency?

your baby. The disadvantages are the cost and the fact that there are few private midwives working outside the large cities.

For further information and to find out whether there is a private midwife in your area write to the Association of Radical Midwives or the Independent Midwives Association (see page 204).

HOME VERSUS HOSPITAL

Home

- You are free to move around and adopt any position you wish for the birth.
- In familiar surroundings you may be more relaxed and so need less, or no, pain relief.
- Birth is a family event. Your other children can greet the new arrival soon after birth or may even be present at the birth.
- You are likely to avoid unnecessary intervention during the process of labour.
- You don't have to worry about getting to the hospital once you are in labour.
- You will be delivered by the same midwife or one of the team of midwives you have had looking after you during your pregnancy.
- You can breast-feed straight away – and on demand.
- You may find it difficult to get enough rest.

Hospital

- You have experts on hand should anything go wrong.
- You won't have to worry about preparing meals and running the home immediately after your baby is born, so you can concentrate totally on being a mother.
- Experts in postnatal care give you advice, which is particularly useful if you have no previous experience of babies.
- You have the company of other new mothers in the same situation, and may even make lifelong friends.
- You may experience more intervention during labour. Afterwards there may be ward routines to conform to which may make it hard to relax.
- You may need more pain relief as a result of being on 'foreign territory'.
- Hospital staff will look after your baby if you need extra rest.

Add any considerations that seem important to you.

....
....
....

PRIVATE HOSPITALS

If you have the money you may like to consider a private hospital. Certainly the hotel side of your care – your accommodation, food, and so on – is likely to be of a higher standard than that in a National Health hospital. As for your medical care, chances are that this will be from an obstetrician who also operates in the NHS, so the treatment you have will depend on his or her views and policies. It's worth finding out what these are before making your booking.

An alternative option is to book an amenity bed in an NHS hospital. You pay a small sum per night, which is about the price of a bed and breakfast in a guest house, for a private room off the main maternity ward. The advantage is that you have full hospital care, plus the privacy of your own room, so you are less likely to be disturbed by other people's babies and ward routines.

How to arrange a home delivery

Once you have chosen a home birth and made sure your doctor is in agreement with your choice, you need to know whether your doctor does home deliveries. If not, he or she should be able to refer you to another doctor in the area who will take you on for the course of your pregnancy and birth. Alternatively you can find the names of doctors specializing in obstetrics from your Family Practitioner Committee or Community Health Council. If your GP is unable to refer you to another doctor or you can't find one yourself you will need to write to the Director of Nursing Services (Community Midwifery) at your District Health Authority, stating your intention of having your baby at home and asking for a midwife to be provided. Send a copy of the letter to the District Medical Officer and Chairman of the District Health Authority. You'll find the addresses in your local telephone directory.

You will then be allocated a midwife, who can call on a doctor should any complications arise during labour.

If you need further help, support or information write to one of the birth organizations (see page 203 for addresses).

Getting the best out of your hospital

The choice of hospital depends generally on the area in which you live. In some areas you may have no choice and in others, particularly in large cities, there may be several hospitals from which to choose. Even with a wide choice, you will probably opt for the hospital nearest your home.

However, if you fall into a high-risk category you may be booked into a teaching hospital or one with the extra facilities necessary to provide for you and your baby should the need arise.

Even if you are booked into the only hospital in your area, you'll want to choose the consultant whose ideas are closest to your own. To find out about the ideas and policies of the different consultants, ask women in your area who have recently had babies. A local birth group may be able to help you by putting you in touch with new mothers. Alternatively, ask around at work or among your friends. Your doctor and midwife may also be good sources of information.

WORKING OUT YOUR BIRTH OPTIONS

It is difficult to decide early on in pregnancy the sort of birth you would like, while you are still coming to terms with the fact that you are pregnant at all. However, you need to give some thought to the matter in order to find the hospital/consultant who suits you. Below is a brief outline of some of the terms used and the issues to consider. You will find these described in more detail in the section on labour.

Natural birth The term natural birth describes an approach towards childbirth rather than a rigid set of rules on the best way to go about it. It rests on the belief that, for most women, birth is a normal process that works best if allowed to progress unimpeded by artificial interference. Medical procedures that are said to alter the natural rhythm of labour are avoided, and instead each woman is encouraged to become attuned to her own body, so as to work with nature rather than against it. Natural birth supporters argue that a 'chain of intervention' is frequently established in labour wards, in which one medical procedure leads to another, resulting in a highly artificial delivery. For example, being started off artificially (induced), means you have to be continuously monitored electronically. This in turn impedes free movement, leading to greater need for chemical pain relief. Because labour is speeded up, and you are not allowed to adopt an upright position, the tissues of the birth canal may not stretch sufficiently, so that a cut (episiotomy) is necessary to make extra room for the baby to be born. Natural childbirth supporters prefer to use techniques such as breathing awareness, relaxation, change of posture and sometimes herbal or homoeopathic remedies to help labour to progress as easily as possible. There's no one way to give birth naturally, but some of the most important influences on natural birth supporters are described below.

Active birth This is a method of giving birth pioneered by birth teacher, Janet Balaskas, and the French doctor, Michel Odent (see below). The idea is that a woman in labour is an active birth giver, rather than a passive patient. During an active birth you move around freely in the way that seems best to you. Keeping mobile enables contractions (the tightenings of the uterus during labour, which open up the cervix and push the baby out) to be more effective. This means that labour is shorter. An upright position enables a good circulation to the baby to be maintainèd, and encourages the baby to rotate into the most favourable position for birth. Gravity aids the baby's descent, and giving birth in a squatting or kneeling position increases the size of the pelvic outlet, so cutting down the need for an episiotomy or caesarean.

Most obstetricians agree that labour progresses more smoothly if a woman is allowed to remain upright. Some hospitals have attempted to cater for this by introducing special birth aids such as the 'birthing bed'. This looks just like an ordinary bed, but it can be converted to allow you to adopt an upright, supported squatting position for birth. However, most active birth supporters would argue that such artificial aids are unnecessary. Simpler aids include a horseshoe-shaped stool on which you can sit to give birth.

Michel Odent Michel Odent is a French surgeon who has been extremely influential within the natural childbirth movement. He believes that women should be allowed to follow their instincts during labour, but that many accepted practices discourage them from doing so. At his hospital in Pithiviers, northern France, Odent created a special 'primitive room' designed to encourage women to follow these instincts. Instead of the conventional delivery bed, it was furnished with cushions, bean bags and mattresses, to encourage women to adopt different positions rather than lying down. He discovered that many women find a warm bath especially soothing and relaxing during labour, and several women found it so effective they didn't want to leave the bath and ended up giving birth underwater! Such 'water births' are perfectly safe as the baby is supplied with oxygen by the umbilical cord, and only starts to breathe as she surfaces. Odent now lives and works with independent midwives in Great Britain, delivering women at home.

Leboyer birth Frenchman Frederick Leboyer popularized the idea that a baby's feelings should be taken into account during birth. His belief that a baby should be delivered into a calm, quiet, unstressed environment has led to his ideas being labelled 'gentle birth'. Lights are dimmed in the delivery room and noise kept to a minimum so as to avoid bombarding the baby with harsh sensations. The baby is delivered on to her mother's abdomen, and her cord is allowed to stop pulsating naturally before being cut. The argument is that the baby gets an extra transfusion of blood, and is not deprived of her former lifeline until breathing is established. After birth the baby is given a tepid bath, said to calm and soothe her by mimicking the watery environment of the womb. Few hospitals practise all these procedures, but many have incorporated gentle birth ideas into delivery. If you would like to have your baby in this way, you can ask to have it written on your notes.

High-tech birth Just as natural birth refers to an approach rather than a method, so high-tech is a shorthand for a particular outlook. The idea behind this is that nature can be unpredictable. Controlling labour by medical methods, it is argued, reduces the chances of things going wrong. Several obstetric techniques are commonly adopted to this end. These are listed briefly here. You will find fuller explanations in the part of the book dealing with labour and birth.

Induction Starting off labour artificially by the use of chemical substances, such as artificial hormones, or physically by stretching the cervix (sweep) or breaking the waters.

Acceleration/augmentation This refers to the use of a hormone drip to control the speed at which labour progresses.

Fetal monitoring The use of equipment capable of picking up the baby's heart rate and the action of your uterus during labour. This is then fed into a computer, which prints out the result. This enables staff to keep a close watch on how well your baby is coping with labour. Monitoring may be continuous, i.e. you are attached to the monitor the whole time, in which case you won't be able to move around much; or intermittent, when the monitor is applied at regular intervals to check on the baby's well-being. When you are not attached to the monitor you are able to move around freely.

Breaking the waters This may be done as part of an induction, or in order to attach an electrode clip or screw to your baby's head for monitoring purposes. It can be a way of speeding up a labour which is going slowly. However, once the waters have been broken most doctors prefer birth to take place within certain time limits (usually 12 hours), because of the risk of infection. If it doesn't, labour may be speeded up or a caesarean may be performed.

Intravenous drip A fine tube is passed into a vein and attached to a drip so that drugs and fluids can be fed directly into your blood stream. These include hormones to stimulate labour, glucose if you are short of energy, fluids if you are becoming dehydrated, and some pain-relieving drugs.

Pain-killing drugs An epidural, in which an anaesthetic drug administered into a space in your spinal column provides complete pain relief during labour. However, staff shortages have meant that an epidural service may not be available on a 24-hour basis in some hospitals. Other commonly used drugs that dull or alleviate pain are pethidine, and gas and air, which you inhale through a mask (see pages 134–8 for the pros and cons of these).

Episiotomy A small cut which is made in the tissues between the vagina and anus to enlarge the birth entrance.

Caesarean section The baby is born through a surgical cut in the abdomen rather than through the vagina. A caesarean may be performed if labour is not progressing, if your baby is becoming short of oxygen (distressed), and more often today if a baby is breech (lying bottom down). Other reasons are listed on page 148.

There are certain other procedures which may be followed without such definite indications of their value. Not all hospitals carry out these practices, but it is as well to be aware of them.

Shaving At one time it was routine to shave off pubic hair on admission to hospital, the theory being that this reduced the risk of infection. This often produced much discomfort after birth. Recent studies have shown that shaving has no effect on infection, and may even, by producing nicks in the skin, increase the chances of it developing. Today shaving is much less common.

Enema An enema or suppositories used to be given to clear out the bowel, so as to avoid involuntary soiling during birth. Research showed that this was unnecessary, and that labour was less painful for women who hadn't had their bowels emptied artificially. There's no need for an enema or suppository if you have recently had a bowel motion, and most hospitals have abandoned the practice.

Confinement to bed In many hospitals you will be put to bed when you go into labour, despite the fact that women are often more comfortable moving about and altering position during labour. However, if you have an epidural, or pain-killing drugs, you won't be able to move around freely.

Privacy Even if you have your own delivery room, staff may come and go without knocking. You may be looked after by many different members of staff, including student nurses or doctors. If you would prefer a more intimate environment you can specify this on your birth plan (see page 45). Dimming the lights, taking something from home, or playing music can all help you create your own private space. Some hospitals provide one or two special birthing rooms, fitted out like an ordinary bedroom with no equipment on display to make the atmosphere more homely.

Companionship Your husband will be encouraged to keep you company during labour in most hospitals today. However, not all husbands want to be there during labour, and you might prefer to have a woman friend, relative, or birth teacher with you instead of or as well as your husband. Studies have shown that having a trusted companion with you during labour can result in a shorter labour and easier birth.

Transfer to the delivery room Although this is becoming less common, some hospitals still transfer women to a different room at the beginning of the second (pushing) stage of labour. Unless there is a special reason for this (e.g. you need a caesarean) such a transfer may be unnecessarily disrupting and increase the chance of cross-infection.

Pushing to order It's common for staff to cheer women on in the second stage or to exert greater pushing effort. Although it can be encouraging to know how you are doing, prolonged straining and holding the breath can be exhausting for both mother and baby. Many experts now believe that the second stage should be allowed to proceed naturally without rigid time limits being set on it. Research shows that it is best to follow your own natural instincts, and that this results in fewer episiotomies and babies born in better condition.

Position for delivery Birth is more efficient if you are semi-vertical, so that gravity can help the baby's descent. However, in some hospitals you may be encouraged to lie on your back, for no better reason than the convenience of the staff. Pushing from a horizontal position not only tends to prolong the second stage, it can also result in a greater need for an episiotomy or forceps delivery.

All of these procedures have a place when properly used. If you need them, a thorough explanation of what is being done and the reasons for it should be given. If your baby is small or unwell these procedures can literally be life-saving. However, in some cases they are used as a matter of routine. Provided you and your baby are well there is no reason why you shouldn't decide whether you would feel happier with a natural or high-tech approach. Are you the sort of person who feels more secure surrounded by all the paraphernalia of high technology? Or do you feel safer relying on your own resources? Other factors, such as the way your baby is lying in the womb (presenting – see page 113), will affect the sort of birth you have. And of course the ideas and views of those caring for you will also play a part. You can use the following checklist to find out more about practices at your hospital, so that you are able to reach decisions about the sort of birth you would prefer, based on full information about the choices available.

If you don't know the answers to the questions below, ask next time you go for an antenatal. Alternatively you may like to make an appointment with the director of midwifery or your consultant to discuss them.

BIRTH CHECKLIST

Labour and birth

- Will my husband be able to stay with me throughout labour?
- What is hospital policy on having another companion present during labour?
- Will I be monitored continuously or at intervals?
- Can I give birth in a squatting, kneeling or alternative position if I wish?
- Does the hospital have any aids such as a birthing bed, stool, pool, and so on?
- How many women have an episiotomy in the hospital?
- If I need a caesarean will it be possible to have an epidural if I wish?
- Will my husband be able to be present during a caesarean?
- What is the induction rate at this hospital?
- What procedures are routinely carried out, e.g. shaving, enema, monitoring? (Many hospitals have now given up shaving and enemas.)
- What pain relief is available? If I choose to have an epidural, will an anaesthetist be on duty day and night to administer it?
- Will a time limit be set on any stage of my labour?

Postnatally

- Can the baby stay with me day and night if I wish?
- How many women leave hospital breast-feeding?
- What policies are there regarding breast-feeding, e.g. will I be able to put the baby to my breast on the delivery bed if I wish and is feeding truly 'on demand'?
- What are the visiting arrangements?
- Is there a special care baby unit?
- If my baby has to go into special care will I be able to be involved in looking after her?
- If my baby is premature will I be encouraged to feed her with breast milk which I have pumped off by hand or machine if I wish (see pages 153–4)?
- If all is well, can I arrange to go home after 24 to 48 hours if I wish?

BIRTH PLAN

A birth plan is a written statement outlining your preferences for your labour and delivery. Some hospitals have a special form on which you can express your wishes. A midwife will go over it with you on one of your visits to the hospital, and it is then attached to your notes. Such a plan is bound to be provisional, as you can't calculate exactly how your labour will progress. So be flexible and prepared to adapt to the situation. However, a written plan can help to focus your attention on the things that matter to you and your husband.

Some mothers-to-be draw up their own plan. If you would like to do this it may be useful to arrange a hospital appointment with a senior midwife, in order to discuss your wishes and ensure they are written on your notes.

Some hospitals dislike the idea of birth plans, as they consider them to be rigid and inflexible, given that labour is an unknown quantity. If you have attendants whom you trust, and can communicate with, you have a better chance that your wishes will be respected, as far as is safely possible once you are in labour. In this case a written birth plan may be unnecessary. However, where you are looked after by many different people a birth plan may be the best way to ensure that whoever cares for you in labour knows your choices. Many of the schemes designed to increase continuity of care during pregnancy and birth enable you to have the same team of midwives looking after you throughout, thus increasing the chances of building up a good relationship with those who are caring for you.

Even if you don't make a written plan, it is a good idea early in your pregnancy to discuss your hopes and wishes with your husband or whoever is going to be with you during labour. Once you are in labour you may not feel much like talking and will rely on that person to interpret your wishes and act as a go-between with the midwife or doctor.

How to make your wishes known to the staff

A birth plan is one way of recording the ways in which you would like your maternity care to be conducted, and it can be useful in helping you to focus on your wishes and gain confidence. However, a written plan is no substitute for talking to those who are caring for you and building up a good working relationship with them.

If you are having your baby in a big hospital, shifts and rotas can make it difficult to build up the sort of staff continuity that ensures trust and easy communication. This, together with the fact that women having babies sometimes feel cowed by those in authority, has led some birth teachers to include assertiveness skills as part of their antenatal training.

As a mother-to-be you are in the unique position of being a patient without being ill. After all, pregnancy is an entirely normal process in most cases. Some women are quite happy to be processed through the system, but many, looking back on the experience, feel that much was done simply as a routine and that they weren't treated as individuals.

Learning how to say and get what you want, within reason, can make the experience much more satisfying. Being assertive doesn't mean being aggressive, nor does it mean having things your own way all the time. It's a way of communicating that ensures your wishes are made plain and are taken into account.

Assertiveness means:

- Learning how to refuse what someone is offering without feeling guilty.
- Learning how to make direct, specific requests.
- Learning how to deal with emotions, such as fear, anger and anxiety, in a constructive way.

It sounds easy enough! But most of us have been brought up to be 'nice' and not to offend people, and it can come hard to start dealing with others in a more direct way, especially if they expect us to be compliant.

There's a world of difference in the way a staff member may give information about, say, a shave or enema. For instance, one may say, 'How do you feel about having a shave?' Another may proclaim, 'I'm just going to give you a shave now, all right?' The first offers you a way of making your own views known, the second deprives you of any real choice. Being aware of such distinctions can help you deal with them if they arise.

No one is suggesting you refuse medically necessary intervention, where the safety of your baby is at stake. But learning to ask for what you want can help you to receive a more personalized service, which ultimately is best for you and your baby.

PREGNANCY

HOW TO HAVE THE BIRTH YOU WANT

Before the birth

- Make sure you are well informed.
- Choose the place of birth carefully.
- Outline your preferences beforehand, using a birth plan if you like.

In hospital

- Explain, or get your husband or other labour companion to explain, what you want.
- Be persistent.
- Be positive. Praise where possible rather than blame. Assume that the staff mean well; it's just that sometimes their attitude is different from yours.
- Be specific. Spell out what you want: not 'I want a natural birth', which is open to all sorts of interpretations, but 'I'd like to be able to move around

COUNTDOWN TO A HOME BIRTH

5. As soon as pregnancy is confirmed
Read the checklist on page 36 to see whether you are suitable for a home birth, or whether it would be more appropriate to have your baby in hospital. If you fall into a low-risk group and you think you'd like a home birth, find out the details from your doctor.

If you like the idea of an active birth, start stretching now. There are several good books and tapes available on the subject, or you can join an active birth class (see page 77).

4. Two to six weeks pregnant
Start planning your home birth now. You can have care from your GP and midwife, a midwife alone (if you can't find a GP willing to attend your birth), or a private midwife. (For private midwives see page 204 for address.)

3. Seven months pregnant
If you haven't already done so, start attending antenatal classes now.

2. Six weeks before the birth
Your midwife will call on you to bring a sterile pack, which she will leave with you to be opened on the day you have your baby.
Gather together the following things:

For yourself
Old nightie, T-shirt, pyjama top
Shawl or cardigan

For the midwife
Two new plastic washing-up bowls
Soap dish

freely during labour' or 'I want to be able to choose the sort of pain relief I have, when I feel the need for it'.
- Be realistic. Realize that labour is uncharted territory: you may change your mind, or circumstances may arise that make it necessary for your 'plan' to be changed.
- Be flexible.

After the birth
- Write to the hospital explaining what you liked and didn't like about your care. This will help other mothers.

Incidentally, when dealing with the staff, sit up straight and look them in the eyes – it's impossible to be assertive when you're lying on your back with your legs in the air! Speak clearly and don't shout or whisper. Maintain eye contact. Don't be afraid to ask for clarification if you haven't understood what has been said to you or to spell out what you want if you disagree.

Long socks (your feet may get cold during labour)
Toilet things
Two or three nursing bras
Nipple cream
Something pretty to change into when you've had your baby
Sanitary towels
Chamber pot
Hot-water bottle
Other comfort aids as suggested on page 93

For the birth
Clean, old sheets for the bed
Waterproof sheet to protect mattress
Convector heater or other background heating
Good light such as angle-poise lamp
Extra chairs and cushions
Foam wedge for use during labour

Nailbrush in clean jam jar
Large plastic jug
Two kettles (for sterile water)
Two buckets with lids
Trolley or small table for equipment

For the baby
Soft, clean towel to wrap the baby in
Layette
Crib or carrycot
Two face cloths
Soap, baby cream, lotion
Baby bath or washing-up bowl
Other equipment as pages 94–7

1. On the day
Phone the midwife as soon as you start having contractions. She will probably visit you to confirm that labour has started. Once you are in established labour, she will stay with you until the baby is born.

Feeding

Spend some time thinking about how you would like to feed your baby. Breast milk has important health benefits for babies. However, if you do not like the idea, or if there are other reasons why you choose not to breast-feed, bottle-feeding can be a good alternative. Although a lot of emphasis is placed, quite rightly, on the benefits of breast-feeding, it is better to bottle-feed with love and affection than to breast-feed through gritted teeth. It has been observed by one feeding expert that, after all, the main aim of infant feeding is to feed the infant! The whole subject of breast- and bottle-feeding is one that is often emotionally loaded. However, you should do what you feel is right for you and your baby, in the knowledge that so long as you observe a few simple rules your baby will thrive no matter how you choose to feed him.

Why breast-feed?

- If you like the idea there is no doubt that breast-feeding is best for your baby's health and well-being. Breast milk has evolved to suit the growth and development needs of human babies. Artificial milks have to be extensively modified in order to make them suitable to be fed to babies. In particular the protein in human milk is specially composed to meet the needs of the baby's growing brain. The fats in human milk are of a type that are readily absorbed and protect the growth of the brain and nervous system. The vitamins and minerals in breast milk are in exactly the right proportions. And scientists are still discovering traces of ingredients that are known to be vital for human growth.
- The composition of breast milk is perfect for your baby. It changes over the course of time to meet a baby's changing needs.
- Breast-feeding protects your baby from infection by preventing the growth of dangerous bacteria in the gut. It also contains antibodies which actively protect your baby from many infectious diseases that you have developed an immunity to.
- Breast-fed babies are less likely to develop allergies. It is thought that 'foreign' proteins in the early days of life can cause a baby to become sensitized, so that when he later encounters that substance he suffers an allergic reaction. Much research is still being carried out into this aspect of breast-feeding.

- There are long-term benefits from breast-feeding too. People who were breast-fed as babies are less susceptible to heart disease and digestive disorders when they get older, although of course there are many other factors that influence the development of these illnesses.
- Breast milk is thought to affect the baby's natural appetite-controlling mechanism, by changes in composition during the course of a feed. This is one explanation given for the fact that breast-fed babies are less likely to become overweight.
- Breast-feeding automatically provides the physical contact and comfort that all babies need to thrive.
- Breast-feeding is cheaper than bottle-feeding. Apart from the cost of nursing bras, and perhaps breast pads, it is free.
- Breast milk is the ultimate convenience food. It is always available at the right temperature whenever your baby is hungry.
- Breast-fed babies' bowel movements smell more pleasant than those of a bottle-fed baby.
- Breast-fed babies suffer less tooth decay than bottle-fed babies, and the sucking action of breast-feeding leads to better jaw development and fewer dental problems in later life.
- Breast-fed babies never get constipated in the way that bottle-fed babies sometimes do.
- Once any initial problems have been overcome, breast-feeding is less time-consuming than bottle-feeding. There's no messy preparation and once your milk supply is well-established a breast-feed can be over within eight minutes, which is useful if you are in a hurry. Of course there will probably be occasions when you want to linger over a feed, because breast-feeding is enjoyable for you and your baby.
- The hormones released during breast-feeding help your womb to shrink back to its normal size quickly. The same hormones are responsible for delaying the return of your periods – although not necessarily your fertility. This can be a boon if you've previously suffered difficult or painful periods.
- Breast-feeding uses up the fat stores laid down in pregnancy, and so helps your figure to return to normal.

WHY BOTTLE-FEED?

Despite the undoubted health advantages of breast-feeding it doesn't always work out for everyone and fortunately bottle-feeding provides a safe option for mothers who can't or don't want to breast-feed.

- Some mothers find the idea of breast-feeding physically repulsive. Others encounter so many problems that it becomes a miserable chore. Babies are very sensitive to such messages, and these feelings may be communicated to your baby because emotions have a powerful effect on the milk-flow mechanism. If you feel really put off by the idea of breast-feeding, it may not be the best way to feed your baby.
- If you bottle-feed, your husband and other people will be able to feed your baby. If you lead a very active work or social life this may be an important factor. Of course, your husband can help play his part in looking after your baby in other ways and, if you decide to breast-feed, he can even give the occasional bottle of breast milk which you have drawn off by hand or pump.
- Some mothers feel very overwhelmed by the total responsibility of a new baby. Bottle-feeding may be a way of off-loading some of the burden. However, you won't know how you feel in advance, so if you think you would like to give breast-feeding a try, remember you can change quite easily to bottle-feeding.
- If you have to take drugs for a chronic illness or medical condition, breast-feeding may be inadvisable. Most drugs pass through in breast milk, but many are safe in the amounts in which they do so. However, some drugs, for example anti-depressants or some kinds used for the treatment of epilepsy, can be harmful. If you really want to breast-feed there are many acceptable alternative drugs for breast-feeding mothers. But you will need to discuss this with your medical adviser before you have your baby.
- Some forms of mental handicap or physical deformity in the baby, such as cleft palate, can make breast-feeding difficult or impossible. There are a number of handicap organizations that can give advice to mothers in such circumstances. The paediatrician at the hospital should also be able to offer help.
- In certain rare cases a baby who is ill may not thrive on breast milk. An example is intolerance of the sugar found in milk. In this case a milk substitute will have to be found.
- Sometimes, despite all your efforts, a baby fails to gain weight. There are simple solutions to this problem (see page 165). But if, having tried to rectify the problem, your baby still seems

unhappy with breast-feeding or you are finding it a struggle, it may be better to give in gracefully. In this case you can rest assured that for however long you managed to breast-feed you have given your baby an excellent start in life.

How will I feed?

How you choose to feed will depend to some extent on your temperament and lifestyle. If despite reading the reasons outlined above you still can't decide how to feed, it may help to work through the following checklist. You can do this either on your own or with your husband, a friend, or a counsellor who has been trained to help breast-feeding mothers (see organizations listed on page 203).

- How were you fed yourself as a baby? What messages did you get from your own mother about breast-feeding?
- How was your husband fed as a baby? How does your mother-in-law feel about it?
- What are your husband's feelings and attitudes towards feeding methods?
- How do you feel when you see a baby being breast-fed?
- How do you feel when you see a baby being bottle-fed?
- What changes have taken place in your breasts? How do you feel about them?
- Do you know anyone who is breast-feeding? Has she encountered any problems? If so, how did she overcome them?
- If you already have a child or children, how did you feed them?
- If you tried to breast-feed but didn't succeed, what went wrong?
- Will you have help in the home after you have had your baby?
- Do you lead a very busy or active life? How would breast- or bottle-feeding fit in?
- Are you a very organized person? How important to you is it that life remains reasonably predictable and organized after the baby's birth?

PREPARING TO BREAST-FEED

During pregnancy the fatty tissue that normally makes up most of your breasts is temporarily replaced with a complex network of ducts and milk-producing cells. There is also an increase in blood flow to your breasts. You may experience tingling and extra sensitivity, and you may notice that the darker area around the nipple, the areola, has become pigmented. Small nodules called Montgomery's tubercles appear too; they secrete lubrication to keep the nipples soft and supple. This is your body's way of preparing you to breast-feed.

In order to breast-feed, the nipple, which has some 15 to 20 openings through which the milk spurts, should stand out well from the surrounding tissue when you are cold or when it is stimulated. If the nipple is flat, or turns inwards (inverted), your baby's sucking will usually draw it out after birth. However, breast-feeding may take extra perseverance in this case. You can improve flat or inverted nipples during pregnancy by wearing a special breast shield, made of plastic with a hole in it, which exerts firm painless pressure around the nipple and helps to draw it out. You can also gently stretch the skin on either side and above and below your nipples for a couple of minutes every day, to help make them more protractile. The midwife or doctor should examine your breasts when you go for your booking visit, and if necessary will prescribe breast shields. If you have any worries about your ability to breast-feed, now is the time to raise them.

You will need to invest in a couple of good, supportive bras (see clothing, page 79), and/or some nursing bras.

You may receive a wealth of conflicting advice about how to prepare for breast-feeding. In fact, apart from the points mentioned above there is no need for any special preparation. A daily shower will keep your breasts and nipples clean. If you wish you can massage a little body oil or cream into your nipples. But in any case the skin around them produces its own natural oils which keep your nipples well lubricated. Avoid using too much soap on the nipples, as it can be drying.

What to buy

- Stock up on convenience foods and fill your freezer, so that you have plenty of easy-to-prepare meals available for the early days when breast-feeding is time-consuming.
- Buy a couple of small bottles and teats and some sterilizing fluid, just in case you want to express milk to be fed to your baby when you are out. There is no need to get a special sterilizing unit; a clean plastic container will do just as well.
- You may like to invest in a simple hand breast pump, especially if you are planning to leave the baby regularly with someone else, and you want to leave him with a bottle of breast milk.
- Buy a packet of disposable breast pads to soak up leaks. Avoid those with a plastic backing, which can make your nipples soggy and liable to soreness.
- You will need three nursing bras and three nightdresses that open at the front. Go through your wardrobe and see which clothes are suitable for breast-feeding. Separates are easiest to manage.

PREPARING TO BOTTLE-FEED

Even if you are planning to bottle-feed you will still need to care for your breasts during pregnancy, as outlined above. Apart from that, you will need to ensure that you have all the necessary equipment for bottle-feeding.

- Sterilizing unit of your choice, plus fluid if you are choosing a chemical sterilization method
- Six to eight bottles
- Selection of teats with different-sized holes
- Bottle brush
- Graduated jug for measuring
- Long-handled spoon
- Salt
- Knife
- Tin of formula of your choice.

You will find more information about breast- and bottle-feeding on pages 162–73.

LOOKING AFTER YOURSELF

EATING A HEALTHY DIET

Your growing baby relies on you for all the nutrients she needs to help her grow strong and healthy, so it's specially important that you have a good diet, with plenty of vitamins and minerals. You don't have to 'eat for two' when you are pregnant – that way, you would risk becoming overweight – but you need to ensure that the quality of food you eat is good.

If you've previously existed on a diet of convenience foods now is the time to start eating more fresh foods. You'll be surprised at the extra vim and vigour that they give you, and you can be sure that you're doing the very best for your baby.

Eating healthily is not difficult. It's just as easy to chop up a few fresh vegetables for a salad as it is to open a packet. Labour-saving devices such as food processors, microwave ovens and freezers now make eating sensibly more convenient than ever before.

What should you eat?

A simple way to have all the nutrients you need is to plan your diet in terms of food groups, and to ensure that you have some foods from each group every day. Aim for as varied a diet as you can. Experiment with the many new fruits and vegetables that appear in the supermarkets, and you'll find healthy eating is enjoyable as well as good for you.

A healthy diet includes some of each of the following foods:

Proteins – meat, fish, offal, eggs, beans, peas, lentils, nuts, cheese
  2 portions a day
Carbohydrates (starchy foods) – bread, rice, pasta, cereals
  5 portions a day
Dairy produce – milk, cheese, yoghurt, butter
  3–4 helpings a day
Fruit and vegetables – green leafy vegetables, such as cabbage, broccoli, spinach, cress, lettuce, chicory; orange and yellow fruit and vegetables, such as oranges, carrots, apricots; fresh fruit – choose from whatever is in season
  5 or more portions a day

In the last few years there's been an explosion of information about the best diet for health. The following guidelines are designed to help you find your way through the diet maze.

- Don't diet when you are pregnant, except on your doctor's advice, but don't overeat either.
- Eat as much of your food as you can raw. Aim to have at least one salad a day.
- Cut out sugar and sweet biscuits or cakes.
- Restrict the amount of hard fats (found on meat and in dairy produce) in your diet. Instead go for polyunsaturated fats, such as sunflower oil or margarine. Polyunsaturated fats are those that are liquid at room temperature.
- Step up the amount of roughage in your diet. Include wholewheat bread, brown rice and pasta, whole cereals and plenty of fruit and vegetables.
- Make your diet as varied as possible.
- Eat fish once or twice a week.
- Eat small, regular meals. Never skip a meal – it could have adverse effects on your baby.

- Cut convenience foods to the bare minimum.
- Keep meals simple.

A sample day's menu is shown below.

Sample day's menu for a mother-to-be

Breakfast Orange or other fruit juice
Wholewheat cereal or muesli with milk
or Fruit juice and yoghurt
Slice wholewheat toast with polyunsaturated margarine and sugar-free spread or yeast extract
Lunch Jacket potato with cottage cheese, grated Cheddar cheese or egg; green salad; fruit
or Lentil or vegetable soup with wholewheat roll; yoghurt or fresh fruit
or Wholewheat sandwich filled with chopped egg, tuna mayonnaise or cream cheese and chives; fresh or dried fruit
Dinner Wholewheat pasta with bolognese sauce, lentil sauce or fish sauce, topped with grated cheese, mixed salad; fruit
or Grilled lamb chop, new potatoes boiled in their skins, salad or lightly steamed vegetables; fruit or yoghurt
or Lentil or chickpea casserole, brown rice, salad; fruit or yoghurt
or Grilled or baked trout, mackerel, herring, jacket potato with margarine, salad or steamed vegetables; fruit
or Fish pie, topped with mashed potatoes mixed with milk and margarine or butter; fruit
or Stir-fried bean sprouts, sweetcorn, mushrooms, cabbage, onion, with slivers of chicken, unsalted cashew nuts, brown rice; dried fruit salad with custard

---

Snacks

You may find as your bump gets bigger that you are more comfortable eating several small meals a day rather than the conventional three big ones. Healthy snacks include dried fruit, wholewheat bread spread with a sugar-free jam, yeast extract, or other savoury spread, unsalted nuts and raw vegetables. Steer clear of sweets, biscuits, crisps and salted nuts.

Tea and coffee

Many mothers-to-be find they lose the taste for tea and coffee. If you find you still enjoy these drinks and you have previously been a heavy tea or coffee drinker it's sensible to cut down to three to five cups a day. Both tea and coffee can block the body's uptake of certain essential minerals such as iron and zinc, and the caffeine contained in them is a stimulant.

Experiment with some of the herbal teas that are now so widely available. Try camomile, or mixed fruit tea, sweetened with a little honey if you like and served with a twist of lemon. Drink fruit juices – grape and apple are ideal if you find the citrus juices too acid – or drink water. The mineral waters flavoured with lemon or lime are very refreshing.

Any old iron?

At one time, when women had several babies at close intervals and a poor diet, anaemia was a real problem in pregnancy, causing exhaustion and leading to low birth weight and other complications. As a result, all pregnant women were prescribed iron supplements often with folic acid or vitamin C to help absorption.

However, in recent years, studies have shown that in most cases extra iron is not always necessary during pregnancy. Iron taken in the form of iron tablets may be difficult for the body to absorb and can cause constipation, which may already be a problem, or diarrhoea.

How can you tell if you need extra iron? You'll be given a blood test early in pregnancy that measures your haemoglobin level (Hb), which is the quantity and quality of your red blood cells. The red blood cells are responsible for carrying oxygen to your baby. If your Hb level falls below 11g/dl you'll be advised to take an iron supplement to ensure that you do not become anaemic and so deprive your baby of the oxygen he needs.

If you look pale or feel breathless or excessively exhausted you may be suffering from anaemia. A simple blood test will confirm the diagnosis, and if you are found to be anaemic iron tablets will usually be prescribed. There is still some controversy over the matter. Doctors vary in their policy.

If the doctor does not consider iron tablets to be necessary there is no need to worry. Recent research has shown that an excess of iron can be just as damaging as too little: it makes the red blood cells too large to cross the placenta and there is an increased risk of post-partum haemorrhage (bleeding).

The best way to avoid anaemia is to follow a wholesome, varied diet. Eat plenty of iron-rich foods, such as meat, liver, cereals, nuts, dried apricots and oily fish. Iron is absorbed more readily if you mix it with vitamin C, so eat an orange or drink orange juice with your meals.

Iron supplements

You may need an iron supplement if:

- You have had several babies at close intervals.
- You rush around a lot and don't follow a good diet.
- You were run down before you embarked on this pregnancy.
- You drink a lot of tea.
- Your haemoglobin level falls.
- You are a vegetarian or eat a restricted diet.

Food cravings

Many mothers-to-be develop an urge to indulge in a particular kind of food or foods. These are often salty, tart or cold foods. Such cravings are usually harmless, so long as you don't indulge in them to excess or to the exclusion of more nourishing foods. Cravings are often the result of changes in taste which occur in pregnancy – no one knows why. The types of irresistible craving for bizarre items, such as soil or coal, that some pregnant women had in the past (the medical term is pica) are now almost unheard of. They were thought to be the result of the body's attempt to compensate for dietary deficiencies.

How much weight should I gain?

It's impossible to be hard and fast about weight gain during pregnancy as so much depends on your existing weight and height and your metabolism. As a rule of thumb you should aim to gain no more than 12.5 kg (28 lb.) but if you are eating sensibly you shouldn't worry if you gain slightly more or less than this.

Where the weight goes at full-term pregnancy

Baby	3.4 kg (7 lb. 7 oz.)
Placenta (afterbirth)	680 g (1½ lb.)
Amniotic fluid (waters)	800 g (1¾ lb.)
Breasts	450 g (1 lb.)
Uterus (womb)	1.1 kg (2½ lb.)
Extra fluid	2.5 kg (5½ lb.)
Extra fat	3.5 kg (7¾ lb.)
Total	12.4 kg (27½ lb.)

Mothers-to-be who were underweight before their pregnancy are more likely to encounter problems during birth and afterwards. Being overweight can also put a strain on your system and lead to birth complications. Follow the diet guidelines laid out above and you stand a good chance of having a happy, healthy pregnancy and giving birth to a strong, fit baby. Don't diet during pregnancy, and don't go for high-calorie, refined foods in an effort to gain weight. Quality is more important than quantity.

You'll probably find that you gain little weight during the first three months of pregnancy. If you are suffering from morning sickness you may even lose a little. You'll gain most weight (about 60 per cent of the total) during the next four to five months, and it's during this time that you are likely to feel at your hungriest. Weight gain slows down during the last two to three months, and you may even lose a little weight in the last few weeks of pregnancy.

To supplement or not to supplement?

Generally speaking, so long as you are eating a good, varied diet and you remain well, there's no need for any vitamin or mineral supplements during pregnancy. The exception might be iron (see page 58). However, certain mothers-to-be may benefit from a general

VITAMINS AND MINERALS

	Effect on your baby
VITAMIN A	Helps your baby's cells, teeth and bones grow strong and healthy.
VITAMIN B COMPLEX AND FOLIC ACID	Aid growth and development of embryo, build brain cells and nervous system. Important for blood formation and to prevent malformations of nervous system.

multi-vitamin and mineral supplement. See your doctor if any of the following apply to you:

- You are vegetarian, vegan, or eat a severely restricted diet (see below).
- You smoke or drink regularly. Smoking depletes the uptake of vitamin C, and drinking can also cause poor absorption of essential vitamins and minerals.
- You are under a lot of stress, for instance if you have serious money worries, housing problems, a stressful or exhausting job. Undue stress can create a demand for more vitamins C and B, and zinc.
- You were run down before starting your pregnancy, e.g. you were underweight, had one or more babies close together, or were still breast-feeding.
- You've recently had a miscarriage or stillbirth.
- You take regular drugs for a pre-existing medical condition.
- You're in your teens.
- You're expecting twins, triplets or more.
- You are allergic to dairy produce or wheat.
- You have to spend some time in hospital during your pregnancy.

Don't take any supplement without informing your doctor.

Effect on you	Found in
Keeps skin and mucous membranes healthy. Helps build body's defences against infection.	Dairy foods, liver, oily fish, egg yolk, green and yellow vegetables, cooked carrots, parsley, fortified margarine.
Aid digestion, prevent eye and skin disorders, help fight infections, aid protein synthesis, for healthy nervous system and blood cells. If you are a vegan a supplement of B12 is advised – consult your doctor.	Brewer's yeast and yeast extract, whole grains, offal, fish, eggs, nuts, dried fruit, milk, wheatbran, cheese, soya beans, green leafy vegetables, wheatgerm.

VITAMINS AND MINERALS

	Effect on your baby
VITAMIN C	Builds healthy placenta, protects body cells, helps iron absorption.
VITAMIN D	Builds healthy bones and teeth.
VITAMIN E	Aids maintenance and growth of red blood cells and other cell membranes.
CALCIUM	Together with vitamin D, builds healthy bones and teeth.
IRON	Helps formation of red blood cells, nails, bones, skin.
SODIUM AND POTASSIUM	Regulate fluid levels in cells, promote healthy blood, muscles, nerves. Sodium found in amniotic fluid.
MAGNESIUM	Aids utilization of calcium and vitamin C. Helps build healthy blood vessels, heart, muscles, teeth, nerves.
ZINC	Helps growth of baby.
IODINE (only minute amounts necessary)	Regulates thyroid activity and mental development.

Effect on you	Found in
Helps iron absorption, helps fight infection and boosts wound healing.	Oranges, lemons, grapefruit, blackcurrants, green and red peppers, tomatoes, watercress, baked potatoes.
Aids calcium absorption and phosphorus to strengthen bones.	Fortified milk and margarine, dairy foods, spinach, herrings, almonds, liver, soya flower. Metabolized by the skin from sunshine.
Helps healing of wounds. Makes for healthy blood vessels, heart, skin, lungs, nerves and pituitary gland. Reduces cholesterol level in blood.	Wheatgerm, eggs, fruit, nuts, vegetable oils, soya beans, cereals.
Helps build strong bones and teeth, protects nerves, regulates heart and acid/alkaline balance of body.	Cheese, milk, sardines and other fish eaten whole, peanuts, walnuts, soya milk, watercress, molasses.
As for baby.	Meat, liver, eggs, sardines, pulses, wholegrain bread, dried apricots, molasses.
As for baby. Sodium important for increase in circulating blood during pregnancy.	Salt, milk, cheese, molasses, parsley, wheatgerm, dried fruit, bananas.
As for baby.	Meat, poultry, fish, nuts, bran, milk, green vegetables, wholegrain flour, wheatgerm.
Aids metabolism of vitamin A. Helps healing of wounds, digestion of starches, aids healthy blood, heart and sex organs.	Oysters, red meat, liver, seafood, nuts, cheese, ginger, sunflower seeds.
As for baby. Promotes healthy hair, nails, skin, teeth.	Fish, seafood, seaweed.

PREGNANCY

If you are vegetarian
There's no reason why a vegetarian shouldn't have a strong, healthy baby. Many people who are vegetarian for health reasons are especially aware of food values and the importance of good nutrition. Mix and match proteins and carbohydrates to obtain maximum benefit from what you eat. For instance, combine lentils with brown rice, seeds or other grains. It's extra important that you have as varied a diet as possible, that you eat plenty of foods containing iron, zinc and vitamin B12 (see the chart below for sources of these).

If you are a vegan
A vegan may benefit from a supplement of vitamin B12, found mainly in meat products. B12 is added to some yeast extracts and plant milks and is also found in bean sprouts and seaweed. As you don't eat dairy products you'll need to make sure you have calcium (generally found in cheese and milk) from other sources such as nuts and pulses. Vitamin D helps calcium uptake, so get plenty of sunshine and eat fortified margarines and plant milks to ensure you get a good supply.

For further advice contact the Vegan Society (see page 204 for address).

Allergies

If you suffer from hayfever, asthma, eczema or other more vague allergic symptoms sparked off by items in your diet you'll need to be especially careful about what you eat, to ensure that you have sufficient essential nutrients.

If you're allergic to milk products you'll need calcium from other sources, such as dried apricots, almonds, sardines, sesame seeds, soya milk, flour and curd.

If you are allergic to gluten avoid wheat products and choose maize, rice, millet, sago and other cereal flours.

Further information can be found in *Good Food Before Birth* by Catherine Lewis (Unwin Paperbacks).

Since allergies tend to run in families, it's worth trying to prevent them developing in your baby. Follow the hints below:

- Eat a good, wholefood diet.
- Aim to breast-feed if you can. Even one bottle of cow's milk may spark off an allergy in a susceptible baby. Get advice from your midwife or a breast-feeding counsellor (see page 50).
- Avoid any foods you know spark off an allergic reaction such as sneezing, runny nose, stomach cramps, skin irritations and so on.

ALCOHOL

Too much alcohol can be harmful to your unborn baby. Eight out of 10 babies born to mothers who are alcoholics or heavy drinkers develop fetal alcohol syndrome, which causes small head, facial abnormalities such as cleft palate and hare lip, heart and kidney problems and other abnormalities of the limbs and genitals. Such babies will usually have some degree of mental retardation too.

If you're just a social drinker, or perhaps drank a little too much over Christmas before you knew you were pregnant, what is the danger to your baby? The harmful effects of drinking vary, but it's generally thought that you have to drink a lot more than two glasses of wine or spirits, or a pint of beer a day for your baby to be affected. Even so, a recent report in Scotland has shown that babies conceived around the Christmas party season are more likely to be premature (although this may not necessarily be due to alcohol). Some women seem to cope better with alcohol than others, as do babies. Whether or not your baby will be affected seems to depend on the amount you drink and how often you do it, as well as a whole range of factors such as genetic susceptibility, environment, and so on.

As always, the most dangerous time to drink is during the first 12 weeks of pregnancy when your baby's vital organs are forming. The only safe advice is to lay off alcohol altogether. If you were drinking before you knew you were pregnant, try not to worry. It's never too late to start looking after yourself. Concentrate on having a good diet, and plenty of exercise, rest and fresh air.

SMOKING

If you are a heavy smoker (more than 10 cigarettes a day) your baby stands a greater chance of being born early and small, and of suffering problems during the first few weeks of life. Mothers-to-be who smoke are also more likely to suffer miscarriage. If you or your husband smoke your baby is more likely to have coughs, colds and other respiratory infections, as well as being at an increased risk of developing asthma and bronchitis. All are good reasons for you and your husband to give up smoking if you can.

This isn't always easy of course, particularly if you are under a lot of stress. You smoke to relieve the stress and the smoking in turn creates further problems. Worrying about smoking is an additional stress in such circumstances. So what can you do?

As always, the critical time to try to give up smoking or cut down to the absolute minimum is during the first 12 weeks of pregnancy. You'll need all the support and encouragement you can get from those around you, so enlist the help of your family, and tell your midwife what you are trying to do. There are various self-help groups which exist to encourage people who are giving up smoking, so ask your midwife or health visitor if she knows of any locally; or write to ASH, who will provide helpful leaflets on giving up and details of local groups (see page 203 for address).

Smoking may leave you short of certain essential vitamins and minerals, as it depletes the body of vitamins A, B and C, as well as zinc and manganese. Ask your doctor whether you should take a multi-vitamin and mineral supplement. Eat well, increase your consumption of fresh foods, and try to build periods of rest and relaxation into your daily routine.

DRUGS

It's best during pregnancy to avoid all drugs unless they are prescribed by your doctor. If you have to take particular medicines for a medical condition such as diabetes, thyroid conditions, epilepsy or any other chronic complaint, tell your doctor you are planning to have a baby so that he or she can make any necessary adjustment to the dosage, or prescribe an alternative medication.

TRAVEL DURING PREGNANCY

As long as you are fit and well travelling isn't harmful during pregnancy. But do bear in mind that pregnancy is tiring, so avoid long, arduous journeys unless they are absolutely essential. Don't take anti-nausea preparations. Towards the end of pregnancy stay close to home in case you go into labour.

Car You can carry on driving for as long as you feel comfortable. Some women observe that their reactions are slower during pregnancy. If this happens to you, it's best to avoid driving as much as possible. After the seventh month your bump may get in the way, and many women find the seat belt is uncomfortable too. Make yourself comfortable by taking a small cushion to put at the base of your spine. Try to empty your

> *Keeping healthy*
> - Avoid all medication, including over-the-counter remedies such as aspirin, unless prescribed by your doctor.
> - When visiting your doctor for an illness during pregnancy, always remind him or her that you are pregnant and ask about any effects on your baby.
> - If you have a pre-existing medical problem don't discontinue treatment but do discuss it with your doctor.
> - Avoid new drugs or those that have just appeared on the market.
> - Never use leftover drugs or anything that has been prescribed for someone else.
> - Do not smoke marijuana or take any other 'street' drugs during pregnancy.

bladder at regular intervals during long journeys, because there is a greater risk of urinary infection during pregnancy.

Train Travelling by train is probably the most pleasant way of getting from one place to another, as there are toilet and usually buffet facilities at hand. Don't be afraid to ask someone to give up their seat on a crowded train.

Flying Most airlines will not let you fly after the 32nd week of pregnancy, and if you wish to do so you will need a note from your doctor pronouncing you fit. If you have suffered previous miscarriages or have a history of bleeding in early pregnancy, it might be advisable not to fly – ask your doctor for advice. Travelling across time zones also imposes a strain, and is to be avoided if at all possible. Incidentally, if you do intend to fly, check that your health insurance covers you for pregnancy.

EXERCISE DURING PREGNANCY

Exercise can help you feel and stay fit. It promotes a feeling of well-being and enables your body to remain supple, which will help you to stand up to labour better and to recover quickly afterwards – all good reasons to continue exercising sensibly during pregnancy, so long as your pregnancy is straightforward.

The effects of exercise on the baby are complicated. When you exercise, some of the blood supply to the baby is diverted to your organs and muscles. Once you stop exercising everything goes back to normal fairly quickly. So long as you are in good health, this temporary shortage in the blood flow has no detrimental effects. If you are suffering from conditions such as high blood pressure or other pregnancy problems, however, it may be wise to avoid exercise, in order to avoid putting undue extra stress on the baby. You'll probably feel less like exercising as your pregnancy draws to an end. If you normally enjoy regular exercise or sport you can continue with it for as long as you feel comfortable. Any exercise that you enjoy, except dangerous sports, is suitable, provided you follow a few simple rules (see page 69).

If you are starting exercise for the first time during pregnancy, choose something gentle such as swimming, walking, or yoga.

Running If you already run it's perfectly safe to continue. Don't run more than about three kilometres a day, and don't run if the weather is hot and oppressive. Avoid running on hard road surfaces as your ligaments soften during pregnancy, making you more prone to injury.

Dancing This is an ideal form of exercise during pregnancy. Avoid strenuous aerobics and exercises that involve overstretching or that put a strain on your back.

Cycling Using an exercise bicycle may be better than cycling on the road, because of changes in your balance. If you are used to cycling you can usually safely continue. Avoid racing handles as the hunched position you have to adopt to use them can cause backache. Steer clear of town centres and main roads.

Swimming This is the perfect exercise for mothers-to-be. Avoid water that is too hot or too cold and don't engage in competitive swimming.

Weightlifting It is safe to carry on this type of exercise, provided you avoid very heavy weights and free weights, but don't start for the first time during pregnancy.

Yoga Again, this is an ideal exercise, so long as you avoid overstretching. Many active birth classes use yoga-based exercise. Make sure your teacher knows you are pregnant, so that postures can be adapted. Some lying down and standing postures may cause low blood pressure. Stop if you feel faint or dizzy.

Exercise dos and don'ts

- Do tell your doctor before embarking on any exercise programme.
- Do take it easy and stop at once if you feel any pain.
- Do exercise regularly, rather than going in for strenuous occasional sessions. Aim for about three times a week.
- Do take your pulse every 10–15 minutes – if it goes over 140 a minute slow down until it is 90 or under.
- Do give yourself time to warm up and cool down.
- Do relax lying down for 10 minutes after exercising, preferably lying on your left side so as to rest your heart.
- Do eat sensibly. You may need to increase the amount you eat slightly to replace calories lost during exercise.
- Do wear a good bra and supportive shoes when exercising.
- Don't exercise to the point of exhaustion.
- Don't do exercises or sports that demand precise balance and co-ordination, and avoid 'contact' sports such as squash or tennis.
- Don't get too hot.
- Don't exercise for more than an hour at a time.
- Don't have very hot showers or baths, and avoid saunas. Keep baths short – not longer than 15 minutes.
- Don't get dehydrated. Drink whenever you feel thirsty during exercise, and after finishing exercising drink a couple of tumblers of water to replace fluids lost through sweating.
- Don't compete.

STOP EXERCISING IMMEDIATELY YOU GET OUT OF BREATH OR IF YOU EXPERIENCE DIZZINESS, NUMBNESS, PINS AND NEEDLES, PAIN OR BLEEDING. CONSULT YOUR DOCTOR.

PREGNANCY

Exercise and relaxation

- If you like the idea of an active birth (see page 40), practise squatting from early on in pregnancy. At first you may prefer to squat against a wall or with the support of cushions under your bottom. As you get more supple and your muscles become stronger you'll be able to squat with your heels flat on the floor and your weight evenly balanced throughout your whole foot. Press slowly against your thighs to increase the stretch. Squat when you use the phone, whenever you are working at a low level (e.g. taking something out of the oven), playing with your children, watching TV, and so on.
- Roll your neck slowly in a circle to ease tension and help you keep supple.

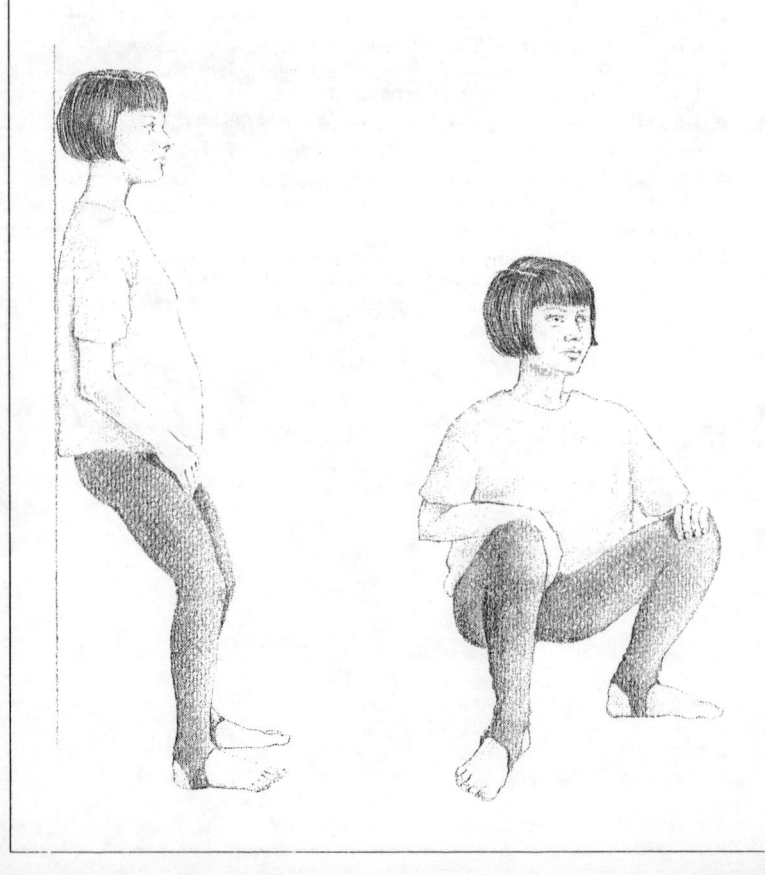

- Practise circling your shoulders to ease tension and improve posture.
- To strengthen your abdomen, lie on a pillow with your legs bent up and your feet flat on the floor. Cross your arms across your abdomen and slowly curl your head and shoulders forward until you are looking at your knees. Then slowly lower head and shoulders. Repeat two or three times a day. **Do not do sit-ups while you are pregnant**.
- Whenever you sit make sure your spine is straight, to avoid backache and putting a strain on your back muscles. Practise by sitting against a wall and pulling your shoulder blades together and down. Press your back flat against the wall for a few seconds.
- To strengthen the buttocks, lie flat on the floor with your knees bent up, feet flat on the floor and arms flat at your sides. Gently raise your buttocks off the floor and twist your hips from side to side. Lower yourself. Repeat two or three times, twice a day.
- To strengthen legs and feet, stand at arm's length from the wall. Step forward on one foot bending at the knee, keeping your back heel flat on the floor. Gently bounce a few times. Then repeat with the other leg in front.
- Practise standing on your toes, then bend at the knees. Repeat several times. Use the back of a chair or the wall for support if necessary.
- Circle your toes in a clockwise and anticlockwise direction whenever you are sitting down, to strengthen your ankles and feet and help the circulation.
- Rest and breathe deeply and evenly after doing any exercise, or after strenuous housework or travel.

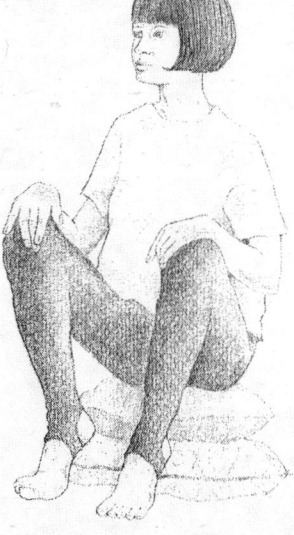

PREGNANCY

Pregnant mothers' instant pick-up

1. Lie on your back and rest your feet against the wall, with straight legs, about 60 cm (2 ft.) above your heart. Place a cushion under your buttocks for comfort if you like. Close your eyes and take a few relaxing breaths.
2. Bring your feet down the wall a little and bend your knees. Now raise and lower your buttocks, pressing against the wall for support and tightening your buttocks and abdomen.
3. Straighten your legs and push up with your hips, so that your body is in a straight line from shoulders to feet. Hold for a few seconds, tightening

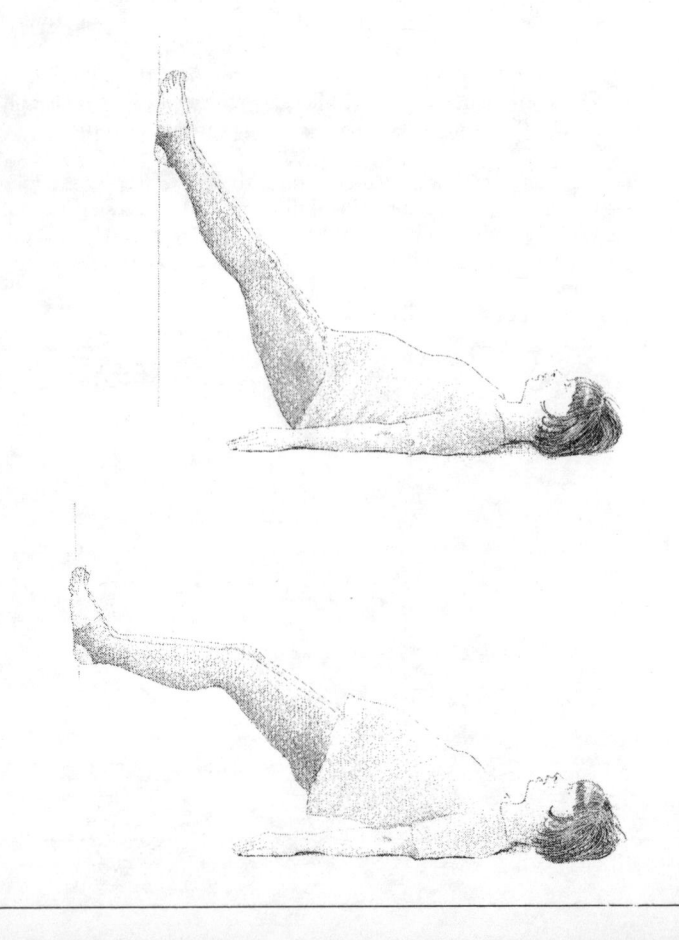

your buttocks to enable you to maintain this position. Repeat a couple of times.
4. Roll gently from side to side, bending first one knee and then the other as you do so.
5. Now lower your legs and bring the soles of your feet together, flopping your thighs apart in the tailor position. Stay like this for a moment or two, relaxing and massaging your thighs to ease any tension.
6. Take three slow deep breaths as you relax. When you feel like getting up, do so slowly by rolling on to your side and then getting on to all fours.
7. S-t-r-e-t-c-h! You'll be amazed at how much brighter you feel.

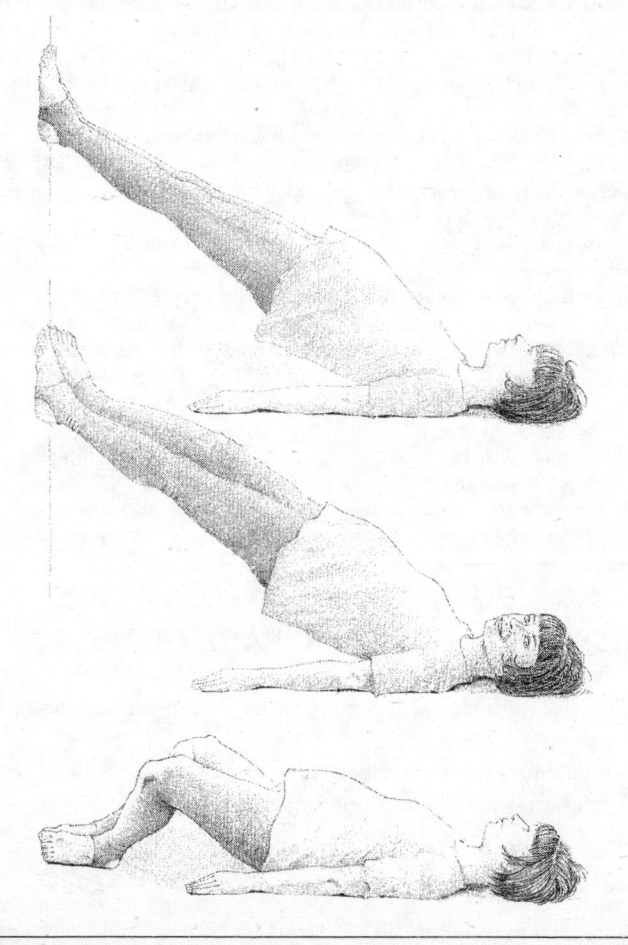

How to relax

There are many techniques to enable you to relax. If this one doesn't suit you, you may find one you prefer in books or cassettes of pregnancy exercises. Alternatively, ask your antenatal teacher to suggest a few methods. Practise relaxing at least twice a day. Once you know how to do it, you can adapt the technique for any time you feel a little tense, for example when waiting for your antenatal, sitting in a traffic jam, and so on.

1. Lie flat on your back with legs bent, feet flat, arms spread and hands open facing the ceiling. If lying on your back is uncomfortable, lie on your side with a pillow under your abdomen and one knee for support.
2. Slowly clench and then completely relax each muscle, moving from the tips of your toes to the top of your head. If you are prone to cramp avoid pointing your toes; instead, flex them upwards before completely relaxing.
3. When you reach your face, grimace as if you were pulling on a tight corset. Then let your face become soft and relaxed, let your mouth drop open slightly, keep your lips soft. Blink a few times and roll your eyes, then softly close your lids.
4. Slowly check back over each muscle group to make sure every part of you is fully relaxed.
5. Now your body is completely relaxed, breathe deeply and calmly, concentrating on each breath in and out. As each thought enters your mind, let it gently float away. You may find it helps to repeat a soothing word or phrase, or count backwards slowly from 100, or imagine a soothing scene, such as a deserted beach or hilltop.

Touch relaxation Practise relaxing as your husband touches each part of your body. Feel yourself soften to his touch.

If you practise relaxing every day you can use the technique during labour, to help counteract any tension.

CLASSES FOR BIRTH PREPARATION

The choice of birth classes depends on what's available in your area and the type of birth you would like.

Classes fall into two basic types: those run by the NHS, and private classes run by a variety of organizations and individuals.

NHS CLASSES

These are held in hospitals, in local health centres, child health clinics

CLASSES FOR BIRTH PREPARATION

and doctors' surgeries. In large hospitals there may be a special antenatal midwife who has responsibility for antenatal classes. She may call on physiotherapists to teach the exercise and relaxation part of the classes, and other specialists such as the 'feeding' sister or the obstetrician. You'll usually be offered a tour of the labour and postnatal wards, so that you are familiar with where you are going to have your baby.

Classes held in other venues are usually run by district midwives and/or health visitors, and a physiotherapist may or may not be involved. If such classes don't include a hospital tour, you should be able to arrange one when you visit the antenatal clinic.

Most classes have at least one session to which fathers are invited, and in a few areas there may be couples' classes. They usually include a birth film and a tour of the unit.

Antenatal classes not only help you to prepare mentally and physically for the birth but provide an opportunity for you to meet other pregnant mothers.

Classes usually start at around the 28th week of pregnancy, and you'll probably be sent a letter telling you when to attend. If you haven't received your notification by the 29th week, mention it to the midwife when you go for your next antenatal check to ensure you don't miss out.

The precise format varies but a typical NHS course is likely to include the following:

- Advice on posture, diet, exercise and adjusting your lifestyle to your pregnancy.
- How your body changes during pregnancy and the way your baby grows.
- Exercise and relaxation techniques to prepare you for labour.
- Breathing techniques to use during labour.
- Signs of labour and when to go to hospital.
- What to expect during labour and what happens when you get to hospital.
- Types of pain relief available and an opportunity to try gas and air equipment.
- Birth film and tour of maternity unit.
- Looking after your baby: pros and cons of breast and bottle, how to bath your baby, how to put on a nappy, and so on.
- Expectant fathers' session.

PRIVATE CLASSES

Classes run by private organizations usually charge a small fee. In genuine cases of hardship, however, the charge will be waived or there may be a trainee teacher in the area who will teach free or for a small donation. Generally, such classes are more detailed and more informal than NHS ones, and there may be more opportunity for discussion.

National Childbirth Trust classes

These classes are held by women who have had children and who have usually taken NCT classes themselves. They may or may not have a medical background (many physiotherapists and midwives go on to train as Trust teachers), but they will all have undertaken the Trust's detailed and searching training, so you can be sure you are in good hands. Classes are usually held in the teacher's own home. Husbands are usually encouraged to attend every class, though some teachers also hold classes for mothers-to-be only, with a single couples' class.

The precise length and content of each course depends on the individual teacher. All the things dealt with in NHS classes are generally covered, though there is less emphasis on baby care. You may get more detailed information about your choices in labour than you would in a hospital class. Classes are usually small, so you get to know the other women or couples who are attending, which, in turn, makes for relaxed and detailed discussion about pregnancy and birth.

Parents who have attended such classes often continue meeting after their babies are born, providing each other with support and friendship in the months and even years after birth.

In many areas, the Trust also has a postnatal support scheme, whereby you are visited by another mother who acts as your personal supporter after you have had your baby and who may take you to coffee mornings and other social activities. Such contact can be invaluable in counteracting feelings of isolation that you may experience in the early weeks of motherhood.

There are also NCT breast-feeding counsellors, mothers who have breast-fed themselves and who have been trained to give non-biased advice and support, either over the phone or in person, if you run into any feeding difficulties.

Classes are popular so book early. For details of your local branch see address on page 203.

Active birth classes

The philosophy behind active birth classes is that birth can and should be a natural event, and that most women are capable of giving birth naturally under the right circumstances. Women attending these classes are encouraged to give birth in an upright or squatting position, which is said to be the most physiologically favourable to a normal, trouble-free birth.

You will be taught a range of yoga-based positions and exercises for use during first and second stage labour, which are designed to make your body supple and give you the best chance for natural birth. You'll be encouraged to start limbering and loosening up early on in pregnancy to enable muscles and limbs unused to strenuous physical exercise to become supple.

Such classes are often attended by women who are interested in the ideas of birth gurus Frederick Leboyer and Michel Odent (see pages 40–41). If you would like to attend such classes contact the Active Birth Movement (see page 203 for address) as soon as you think you may be pregnant. If there isn't an active birth class in your area you may like to buy a book or a tape on the subject (see suggestions on page 205).

Birth Centre classes

At Birth Centres, as at active birth and NCT classes, the emphasis is on natural birth. In order to help you achieve as natural a birth as possible at home or in hospital (and many women who attend Birth Centre classes are committed to home delivery), you will be taught about the importance of good nutrition, alternative remedies for pregnancy ailments and labour, and, if you are having your baby in hospital, ways in which you may be able to avoid unnecessary intervention. This may include the use of assertive techniques to enable you to make sure you have your wishes respected.

For a list of Birth Centres see page 203 for address, and make sure you book early in pregnancy.

MAKING THE MOST OF YOUR APPEARANCE

CLOTHING

The physical changes of pregnancy will affect your choice of clothes. Sweating is increased during pregnancy, and the greater volume of circulating blood that your body produces to provide for your baby, plus your extra weight, means you feel hotter than usual. Light clothes in natural fibres that absorb sweat and keep you feeling and looking cool are most suitable.

For the first four or five months of pregnancy you will probably be able to get by with your ordinary clothes, given one or two small adjustments. Clothes such as dungarees, or those with an elasticated or drawstring waistband, expand along with you and can be used until they are too tight. However, as your bump becomes more prominent you will probably need to invest in one or two maternity outfits. What you buy will depend on your lifestyle. You may need to look smart for work, in which case you should avoid frilly, flowery smocks and go for something more tailored. If you are at home looking after other children, trousers and baggy sweatshirts may well be appropriate.

Think about what the weather is likely to be when you will be at your largest. If your baby is due in the summer you will need light, cool cottons. If he is due in the winter, what are you going to wear outside? A coat is a big investment, but a cape or poncho might be just as good, and you don't have to spend a lot on a garment that will be unsuitable once you stop being pregnant.

If you need clothing for a special occasion, or if your job demands that you need a lot of different outfits, it may be preferable to hire rather than buy. Bumpsadaisy, a maternity-wear shop that operates a hire service, specializes in mail order (see page 204 for address).

Tips on buying and choosing clothes
- Have a look through your wardrobe and set aside anything that can be adapted, such as trousers or skirts with elasticated or drawstring waists, big baggy shirts (raid your husband's wardrobe too), smocks or loose shapes, long cardigans and sweaters. Many clothes can be adapted with a few simple dressmaking techniques such as inserting an elasticated panel.
- Check out ordinary fashion outlets as well as special maternity wear shops for loose jackets, dresses and tops. They are often more up-to-date than conventional maternity clothes. Look in the menswear section too.
- Choose clothes that are loose and unconstricting. Avoid tight waistbands, or anything that is tight around the abdomen or thighs. Your breasts will be bigger, so avoid anything with a tight bodice.

- You will probably need to wear your maternity clothes for a little while after the birth until you get your figure back. If you plan to breast-feed, look for clothes that open down the front.
- Buy clothes that are easy to care for and launder.
- Choose clothes that fit in with your usual style of dressing. There's no need to float round in floral smocks if you normally wouldn't be seen dead in them. And it will be bad for your morale if you do so. If you don't find what you want straight away, persevere.
- Wear support tights and low-heeled shoes. You may need shoes a half size bigger than usual, because of your extra weight and a tendency for the feet to swell.
- It can be boring wearing the same few clothes all the time. Ring the changes by swapping with friends who are pregnant at the same time. Or see if relatives or friends who have had babies have maternity outfits you could borrow.
- To draw attention away from your bump go for clothes which balance your shape and/or emphasize your head and neckline. For instance, shoulder pads, design details at the neck, drop-waisted dresses, boxy jackets. Long clothes such as cardigans, jackets and tunics also disguise the bump. Avoid anything that clings.
- Choose cotton underclothing. Cotton knickers are essential as you have an increase in vaginal discharge during pregnancy. Bikini briefs that don't exert pressure on the bump are better than knickers which are elasticated around the waist.

Choosing a bra

Even if you don't normally wear a bra you need to do so during pregnancy for comfort, and to prevent your breasts from dropping later on. Your breasts increase in size during pregnancy as fatty tissue is replaced by milk-producing glands. Your breasts will remain this size afterwards until you stop breast-feeding, with the exception of the few days after your milk 'comes in', when they will temporarily swell even larger.

- Choose a bra with wide adjustable straps and a broad supportive band under the cups, preferably with an adjustable fastening.
- Make sure the cups fit snugly with no gaping, especially at the armpit.
- Cotton or a cotton mixture will be more comfortable.
- If your breasts are very heavy you may need a light, stretchy sleep bra to wear in bed.

- It is more economical to buy bras which can double as nursing bras when you are breast-feeding. Even if you choose to buy separate bras you should buy a front-fastening, adjustable bra around the 37th week of pregnancy, for use after you have had your baby. If you intend to breast-feed you will need at least three. Avoid the type which has a flap-opening as these can cut into the breast tissue and cause breast infections.
- If you fall outside the usual range of sizes, for instance if your back is very narrow or your breasts are especially big, the National Childbirth Trust (see page 203) produces a good range of bras in almost all sizes. Ring them to find out your nearest fitter.

LOOKING BEAUTIFUL

Pregnancy is traditionally a time when women bloom. It is true that the increase in hormones and other physical changes can lead to your hair and skin looking better than ever before. But some women find that their hormones play havoc with their appearance. For every woman whose skin is supple and glowing, there is one who complains of an increase in spottiness. And while there are many whose hair becomes shiny and manageable, there are a host of others who find it becomes dry and unmanageable. However, there are several beauty tricks which are worth trying to help you look good and feel more comfortable.

Skin The increase in circulation can give the skin a rosy glow. Too much ruddiness can be toned down by smoothing on a green foundation under your usual one.

Pregnancy hormones bring about an increase in skin pigmentation and this may be especially noticeable if you are a brunette or dark-skinned. Some women develop a butterfly-shaped patch of pigmentation across the face, known as chloasma, or the mask of pregnancy. Increases in pigmentation can be intensified by the sun, so choose a foundation that contains UVA filters. Use a concealer stick to disguise any marked areas of pigmentation. Pigmentation will disappear within three months of your baby being born.

Skin can become dry or oily. Use a gentle, hypoallergenic skin care product. If dry skin becomes itchy use plenty of light, easily absorbed moisturizer. A calamine-based cream can also soothe itchiness. If the skin on your abdomen becomes dry, use a rich body lotion or a special pregnancy cream. These won't prevent stretch marks from appearing, as this is caused by the deeper layers of skin tissue becoming overstretched, but they will help you feel more comfortable. Use a bath oil or moisturizing foam bath to pamper yourself and prevent water loss.

Tiredness and fluid retention can lead to puffiness around the face, noticeable under the chin and around your eyes. Soak a couple of pieces of cotton wool in witch hazel and lie down with them over your eyelids for 10 minutes, or use an eye gel, available from leading cosmetic companies. To camouflage a puffy chin, use a darker shade of foundation in that area.

Hair Pregnancy hormones prevent the normal constant shedding of hairs that occurs, with the result that your hair is thicker. You may suddenly lose what seems like an alarming amount of hair three months after delivery when your hormones get back to normal. In the meantime make the most of your thick hair. A good easy-to-care-for cut is a sensible investment, and will stand you in good stead once the baby is born, when you won't have time to manage a fussy hair style. The way hair reacts to hairdressing treatments sometimes alters during pregnancy, so inform your hairdresser that you are pregnant. It's best to go for non-chemical, gentle hair colourings such as henna or camomile during pregnancy rather than harsh bleaches and dyes.

Teeth and gums Bleeding, swollen gums and other dental problems sometimes arise for the first time in pregnancy. Brush your teeth well three times a day. Massage the gums with your finger before brushing, and use a small-headed, soft-bristled toothbrush. Make an appointment to see your dentist. It's free while you are pregnant.

MINOR AILMENTS OF PREGNANCY: AN A–Z

Backache
This is caused by the softening of your ligaments under the influence of pregnancy hormones and by the changes in posture brought about by the extra weight of your bump. Occasionally it can be a sign of a urinary infection that has ascended to your kidneys, so mention it to your doctor, especially if you've had any urinary problems, such as stinging when you pass water.

You can help yourself by wearing low-heeled shoes and making an effort not to hollow your back when standing for any length of time. Have plenty of rest and put a cushion in the small of your back when you sit down. When you get out of a chair, lever yourself forward to the edge so that you avoid heaving yourself up. Sleep on a firm mattress. If your mattress has a hollow in it put a board underneath to make it firmer. Swimming and yoga are excellent exercises that will both strengthen your back muscles and relieve backache.

Breathlessness

You may find you become short of breath when you exert yourself or climb stairs, especially towards the end of pregnancy before your baby has dropped into the pelvis and when your uterus is pressing upwards on to your diaphragm and lungs. Stand or sit up straight and take it easy. Breathlessness is nature's way of forcing you to slow down.

Constipation

The higher levels of the hormone progesterone in your body during pregnancy have the effect of relaxing all your muscles, with the result that your digestive system slows down. Go for a high-fibre diet, including lots of raw fruit and vegetables, and make sure you have plenty to drink. Exercise frequently and allow yourself time to empty your bowels. Don't strain but relax all your pelvic floor muscles (see page 176).

If you are taking iron tablets you may become constipated, so let your doctor know and he or she may be able to change your prescription. If constipation becomes really troublesome the doctor will be able to advise on or prescribe a mild natural laxative.

Cramp

Cramp in the calves and feet is common in late pregnancy and often wakes you up at night in its iron grip. It may be caused by a lack of salt or calcium in your diet. So make sure you're eating sufficient foods containing calcium, such as milk, cheese, nuts, seeds, and so on (see page 62 for other sources), and that you are getting adequate vitamin D – the sunshine vitamin – that enables your body to absorb calcium. If cramp is a real problem the doctor may prescribe a calcium supplement.

To help yourself, hold your toes with your hand and pull them sharply towards you to extend and 'unlock' the calf muscle, or get your husband to massage firmly the affected area. You may find it helps to raise the foot of your bed about 20–25 cm (8–10 in.), by putting blocks or books under the feet. Make up your bed loosely to avoid pressure on your toes and avoid pressing your toes downwards. Practise circling your toes clockwise and anticlockwise to exercise your calf muscles and increase the circulation.

Cystitis

Pressure on the bladder and increased blood flow to the area may make you more susceptible to urinary infections, especially during the early part of pregnancy. The symptoms of cystitis are a burning, stinging sensation when you pass water, a frequent need to pass urine, and perhaps a dull pain in your lower abdomen. Cystitis can become rapidly worse and ascend to your kidneys, so it's important to seek immediate treatment. Your doctor may prescribe a course of antibiotics and a special alkaline solution to neutralize your urine and stop the stinging. In the meantime, drink plenty of fluid (about 300 ml/½ pint every hour). Lemon barley is a good choice as it is alkaline. Rest with a hot-water bottle against your abdomen. You can help prevent further attacks by wearing cotton underwear, and stockings or crotchless tights to allow plenty of circulation of air around the genital area. Make sure you have plenty to drink and don't put off going to the toilet. Always wipe your bottom from front to back to avoid bacteria entering your urethra.

Haemorrhoids (piles)

These are varicose veins of the anus and may be caused by undue straining if you are constipated. Follow the dietary suggestions listed under constipation (above). You can relieve the discomfort by wearing a sanitary pad soaked in witch hazel, or your doctor can prescribe a special cream and stool-softening suppositories. Haemorrhoids usually shrink once you've had your baby.

Heartburn

Late in pregnancy you may tend to regurgitate some 'acid', which causes a stinging sensation in your gullet. Once again, it's the pregnancy hormones that are responsible, together with your baby's increasing size pressing on the stomach. Avoid fatty and spicy foods, and eat small, frequent meals. Try sitting upright for at least 30 minutes after a meal. A drink of warm milk before you go to bed may help, as may sleeping propped up with pillows.

Insomnia

This is often a problem late in pregnancy. It arises partly because it's difficult to get comfy in bed once your bump gets big and your baby is more active, and perhaps because of anxieties concerned with the coming event. Try to give yourself time to wind down in the evening before going to bed. Play some relaxing music, have a meditation or practise your relaxation. Have a warm, soothing bath, adding to it an aromatic oil such as lavender, to help you relax. A warm, milky drink, or camomile tea, will help calm you down. Try sleeping on your side with a pillow under your knee for comfort. Talk about any anxieties and fears you may have with your husband, your midwife or antenatal teacher.

Nausea and vomiting

Nausea is one of the first signs of pregnancy and affects one in two pregnant women. Inaccurately known as morning sickness, since it afflicts many women all through the day, it is caused by high levels of the hormone human chorionic gonadotrophin (HCG), which is circulating in your body during the first three months of pregnancy, and generally passes off at about 12 weeks. Eat small, frequent meals and avoid fatty or spicy foods or anything that you know sparks off the sensation of nausea.

Before getting out of bed in the morning have a dry biscuit or piece of toast and milky tea, or orange or apple juice, and allow yourself plenty of time to get up. Sips of apple or grape juice, or anything else you can take throughout the day, can help stave off the nausea. It usually becomes worse if you have an empty stomach, so carry a small hoard of snacks with you (preferably wholesome ones such as dried or fresh fruit, nuts and wholemeal sandwiches) to nibble on throughout the day. Some women find ginger – either crystallized or a teaspoon of it dissolved in water with a spot of honey to taste – is helpful. If the nausea becomes really bad, lying flat on your back with a hot-water bottle pressed against your abdomen may bring relief. Consult your doctor if the nausea is unusually severe or if sickness persists beyond 16 weeks.

Nosebleeds
You may find your nose is congested so that you feel you have a permanent cold or that you suffer nosebleeds. They are caused by the higher hormone levels softening the mucous membranes throughout your body. Avoid blowing your nose hard.

Thrush
The alkaline-acid balance of your vagina may be disturbed during pregnancy leading to a tendency to thrush, a vaginal yeast infection that produces a thick, white discharge which is unbearably itchy. If you've been treated with antibiotics for cystitis you may be especially prone, since some of these drugs kill off not only the bad bacteria but the good ones too, allowing the yeast to grow. Live natural yoghurt, taken by mouth or placed on a pad against your genitals, may bring relief. Never insert anything in your vagina during pregnancy unless your doctor prescribes pessaries to treat the thrush. Help avoid further attacks by wearing loose, cotton underwear and eating a wholefood diet.

Tingling and numbness of the hands
This is known as the carpal tunnel syndrome and is a result of pressure on the nerves and tendons in your wrist, caused by swelling of the ligaments. Raise your hand above your head for a few moments to drain the fluid and flex your fingers. Occasionally, if the condition is really troublesome, your doctor may prescribe diuretics to ease the swelling.

Tiredness
Towards the end of pregnancy the extra weight of your baby may make you specially tired. Tiredness is often your body's way of forcing you to slow down and shouldn't be ignored. Try to build regular rest periods into your daily routine when you sit with your feet up. Sit outside when the weather is fine and practise deep breathing or your relaxation routine. If you go out to work try to adjust your working hours to avoid the rush hour. If you have other children arrange for them to be looked after now and again by friends or relatives, to give you a break. If your toddler has an afternoon nap take the opportunity to rest too, and have a couple of early nights a week.

Excessive tiredness can be a symptom of anaemia so make sure you have sufficient iron-rich foods in your diet. If you feel constantly tired and nothing seems to help, consult your doctor.

Varicose veins

Again, these are caused by the softening effects of the hormone progesterone and the increased size of your baby, which restricts the circulation return from your legs. You may develop varicose veins in your legs, your anus where they are known as haemorrhoids or piles (see above), or even your vagina. Avoid sitting with your legs crossed, which compresses your veins and causes the blood to collect in your legs. Keep the circulation flowing by getting plenty of exercise, especially walking. When you are sitting practise circling your feet and have plenty of rest with your feet up. Support stockings or tights put on first thing in the morning will prevent your veins overfilling. You may need help with putting them on late in pregnancy when your bump makes it difficult to bend down.

If you develop varicose veins in your vagina a sanitary pad pressed firmly against the veins can bring relief, or an ice pack placed against the tender part is soothing. Lying down with your feet raised helps relieve pressure on the veins, and vitamin B6 tablets are said to help. However, do tell your doctor if you are taking extra vitamins.

Danger signs

Consult your doctor if you develop any of the following:
- Bleeding from the vagina.
- A temperature and general feeling of illness.
- Abdominal pain.
- Severe headache, especially if accompanied by any visual disturbances.

None of these signs is necessarily serious but you should always consult your doctor about them in case they are an indication of a medical condition that needs prompt attention.

MISCARRIAGE

It's thought that about one in five pregnancies ends in miscarriage. Though it's little comfort at the time, it may help to bear in mind that a miscarriage is often nature's way of preventing the birth of an abnormal baby. About 50 per cent of miscarried fetuses are found to be abnormal in some way. Miscarriage can be a result of hormone problems, disease or infection and malnutrition, although a late miscarriage (i.e. one after 12 weeks) is more usually caused by a weak cervix or some abnormality of the uterus.

Bleeding is usually the first symptom, sometimes accompanied by period-type pains. If you start to bleed call the doctor and go to bed. Sometimes the bleeding stops and the pregnancy continues (threatened miscarriage); but if the pain and bleeding increase there is probably nothing you can do to stop miscarrying (inevitable miscarriage).

You may be admitted to hospital, where a D & C (dilatation and curettage) may be performed to clean out your uterus.

After the miscarriage

You may have backache, a vaginal discharge, breast tenderness and, if it was a late miscarriage, you may even produce milk. All these serve as painful reminders of the baby you have lost. Worse than these physical discomforts however, are the misery and guilt you probably feel, and although such emotions are natural, do bear in mind that the miscarriage wasn't your fault.

Before you try again

- Make an appointment to see your doctor for a thorough physical check-up to sort out any problems, such as fibroids, or clear up any infections.
- If your miscarriage was caused by a weak cervix you will probably be able to arrange to have a special stitch put in it during your next pregnancy to prevent another miscarriage.
- Follow a good diet (see page 56) and ask you doctor if you would benefit from a course of vitamins and minerals.
- Cut out drinking and smoking.
- Concentrate on getting yourself in tip-top health. Enrol in an exercise class, make sure you have plenty of rest and relaxation, and sort out any physical problems.
- Use a barrier method of contraception (see page 186) until you are ready to try again.
- Aim to wait three to six months before another pregnancy. It isn't harmful to become pregnant before that but it is useful to give yourself time to recover fully before embarking on the strain of another pregnancy.
- Contact the Miscarriage Association or the National Childbirth Trust, or talk to your doctor or health visitor if you still feel distressed about the miscarriage.
- Remember that most women who have a miscarriage go on to give birth to a normal, healthy baby.

Talk to your doctor or health visitor if the feelings persist, and allow yourself time to work through your grief. It can also help to talk to someone who has had the same experience. The Miscarriage Association is a self-help group, which exists to give support to women who have experienced a miscarriage. Its members have all undergone miscarriages themselves. You'll find the Association's address on page 203.

Will it happen again?

If you have had just one miscarriage you stand an excellent, 80 per cent chance of giving birth to a healthy baby next time. If you have had more than one miscarriage the odds are slightly reduced. The good news is that most women who have had one or more miscarriages eventually carry a baby to term. Even the unfortunate few mothers-to-be who have one miscarriage after another (recurrent miscarriage) usually succeed in the end. It's now thought that recurrent miscarriage may result from the failure of the mother's immune system to 'recognize' her baby, and there are several promising new lines of treatment under investigation.

THE RHESUS FACTOR

Your blood is either Rhesus positive or Rhesus negative. About 85 per cent of people are Rhesus positive, that is their blood contains a substance called the Rhesus factor (a kind of protein antibody stimulant called an antigen). You will be tested to see if you are Rhesus positive or negative on your first visit to the booking clinic. If you are Rhesus positive there is no problem. If you are Rhesus negative and the baby's father is Rhesus positive special precautions need to be taken to avoid the development of a condition known as Rhesus disease in your baby. The Rhesus factor is inherited, so if the baby's father is positive, then the baby could be positive too. Throughout pregnancy small amounts of blood cells from your baby pass into your circulation. At birth, when a large amount of the baby's blood mixes directly with the mother's, a Rhesus negative mother carrying a Rhesus positive baby reacts by producing antibodies against the Rhesus factor.

In a first pregnancy this is not usually a problem, as insufficient of the baby's blood cells pass into your circulation before birth for antibodies to be formed. However, if you are Rhesus negative and you conceive another Rhesus positive baby your body's alarm bells start to ring. The antibodies in your system start to attack the baby's blood cells, causing anaemia, swelling of the liver and spleen, brain damage and even death.

Fortunately today there is much that can be done to prevent this tragic occurrence. Immediately you have given birth to a Rhesus positive baby you can be given an injection of anti-D immunoglobulin, a serum which prevents your body from rushing to attack Rhesus positive blood. The same will happen if you have a miscarriage or termination, and after every baby you have.

If you are Rhesus negative you will have regular blood tests throughout pregnancy to establish whether your body has a high number of antibodies to the Rhesus factor. If it has, your baby could be at risk, and an amniocentesis (see page 29) will be performed so that the waters may be analysed for the presence of bilirubin, a substance produced by the spleen, which indicates that the baby's blood cells are under attack.

If your baby is found to be suffering from Rhesus disease, and is at a stage in pregnancy where it would be safe for her to be born, labour may be induced early. After delivery your baby will need to spend time in special care, and may be given a blood transfusion in order to remove the antibodies from her blood stream, depending on how severely she is affected.

If, however, you baby is too premature to survive were she to be induced, she may need to be given one or more blood transfusions while she is still in the uterus. Thankfully with accurate detection and treatment this is extremely rare today.

Worrying symptoms: what they mean

Bleeding in late pregnancy
Bleeding after 28 weeks of pregnancy is called antepartum haemorrhage. Harmless bleeding may be a result of causes such as cervical erosion – a sore patch on the neck of your womb – or polyps (growths). Nonetheless, if you experience bleeding late in pregnancy you should always call your doctor, as it could be serious. There are two main causes:

Abruptio placenta Sometimes the placenta starts to shear away from the wall of the uterus. You'll bleed from the vagina and may experience pain. No one really knows what causes it, although it often happens if you are suffering from pre-eclampsia (see below) or have raised blood pressure.

The condition can vary from mild to severe. If it is mild you will have no more than a slight trickle of blood from the vagina. You will be admitted to hospital and a blood test will be carried out, you will have a scan to check the position of the placenta and tests to see that your baby is healthy. If all is well with you and the baby, and once the bleeding has stopped, you will probably be allowed to go home. Your pregnancy will then continue as normal, although the obstetrician will want to keep a careful eye on you thereafter and will probably want to induce you (see page 142) if you don't go into labour when you reach your expected date of delivery.

In more severe cases you may need a blood transfusion and your baby will be delivered immediately, probably by caesarean.

Placenta praevia This is when the placenta is embedded so low down in the uterus that it partially or completely blocks the birth outlet. The risk is of severe bleeding when the stronger practice contractions (known as Braxton-Hicks) of late pregnancy begin to draw up the neck of your womb, causing the placenta to start separating from the wall of the uterus.

You'll be admitted to hospital for an ultrasound scan to check the position of the placenta and for tests of your baby's well-being. In mild cases where the placenta is barely lying across the cervix you may be allowed home – so long as your baby is healthy – and advised to get plenty of rest. A normal delivery may be possible, though preparations will be made for an immediate caesarean should it become necessary during labour.

In more severe cases, or if the condition occurs after 38 weeks, the baby will be delivered immediately, usually by caesarean.

Pre-eclampsia

One of the main purposes of your antenatal care is to spot pre-eclampsia, the high blood pressure disease of pregnancy. Pre-eclampsia is insidious because it is a silent disease – symptoms do not appear until the disease has taken hold. There are early signs that can be picked up to show it may be developing. The first signs are protein in the urine and a raised blood pressure. There may also be swelling of the legs, ankles, face and hands due to fluid retention in the tissues, although many pregnant women experience some swelling that isn't serious. Doppler scans (see page 28) can pick out women at risk of developing pre-eclampsia, and later in pregnancy can detect if the baby is receiving enough food and oxygen via the placenta.

Severe pre-eclampsia causes headache, blurred eyesight, dizziness and sickness. If left untreated the placenta begins to fail and may start to separate from the wall of the uterus.

In mild cases of pre-eclampsia the treatment is rest, either in hospital or at home, and occasionally drugs to try to reduce the blood pressure. This careful treatment ensures that pre-eclampsia almost never progresses to actual eclampsia – a severe illness in which fits can result in the death of mother and baby. Regular scans and other checks of fetal well-being will be carried out, and your baby will be delivered as soon as he is strong enough to survive outside the womb. You will usually be given an epidural (see page 135) to lower your blood pressure during labour, and if any complications arise a caesarean will be carried out.

The only treatment in cases of severe pre-eclampsia is immediate delivery of your baby.

A careful eye will be kept on you in the first few days after birth, as the blood pressure can suddenly rise. After this short period of time the condition begins to subside.

Pre-eclampsia is commonest in first pregnancies. It can also run in families, so if your mother suffered from it you may be more prone to developing it. One theory is that it has something to do with the body's failure to 'recognize' the baby as its own, which sets up an immune reaction causing the placenta to be restricted in its growth and function. Usually after one pregnancy your body is geared to recognize any future babies and you'll have no further problems, but about one in 10 women suffer in subsequent pregnancies. Women who are having a baby by a fresh partner and who have previously suffered pre-eclampsia often seem to develop it again – a curious fact that seems to confirm the immune system link.

The hope is that in future it may be possible to prevent pre-eclampsia by 'immunizing' mothers-to-be *before* they become pregnant, in order to persuade their bodies that they have already experienced a pregnancy.

At the moment the main ways in which you can avoid serious problems from developing are by following the healthy pregnancy tips outlined on pages 55–65 and making sure you keep your antenatal appointments. A large-scale trial is taking place to see whether daily low doses of aspirin during pregnancy will prevent the development of pre-eclampsia.

Sugar in the urine

Every time you go for an antenatal check your urine will be tested for glucose. During pregnancy some women develop a type of sugar intolerance known as gestational diabetes. If the sugar level in your urine is continually too high you may be given a glucose tolerance test, which involves testing your urine for glucose after fasting. If the test proves abnormal you will be carefully monitored and may be induced if you haven't gone into labour by the end of pregnancy, to prevent your baby from growing too big. The condition usually subsides once your baby is born.

PREPARING FOR YOUR BABY

A few weeks before your baby is due gather together all the things you will need for your stay in hospital, and make sure you have everything you and your baby will need when you return home (see below).

Now is the time, too, to finish making all those practical, last-minute preparations to smooth the way when you bring your baby home.

- Work out ways of making your home as smooth-running as you can; for instance, if you can afford it, invest in a washing machine, freezer, microwave and other labour-saving devices.
- Work out with your husband how you can share the household chores after your baby is born. You could organize an evening a week when you have a grand clean and tidy together, do a weekly shop at the supermarket, and so on.
- Spring-clean the house if it needs it – but avoid climbing on furniture or ladders.
- Make your house baby-proof. Clear away unnecessary bits and pieces that collect dust, and check the safety of household appliances.

You'll find more tips on safety in *The Mother & Baby Book of Your Baby's First Year.*
- Invest in some extra storage if possible – baby paraphernalia takes up an enormous amount of space!

WHAT TO TAKE INTO HOSPITAL

Comfort aids for labour

- Cotton nightie, T-shirt or loose top if you want or have the choice to wear your own
- Ice cubes in wide-necked vacuum flask
- Apple or grape juice, mineral water
- Honey or glucose sweets to sustain energy
- Small natural sponge to suck on (you dip it in iced water)
- Evian water spray
- Oil or talc for massage
- Flannels, hairbrush and lip salve
- Hot-water bottle
- Socks (the feet often get cold during labour)
- Something to concentrate on, such as a vase of flowers, favourite picture, etc.
- Loaded camera
- Personal stereo or portable tape deck, with a selection of soothing tapes, or a radio
- Books, magazines, packs of cards or games, to while away the time if you have a long labour
- Money for the telephone
- Sandwiches or a snack for your husband or labour companion
- Address book
- Notebook and pen
- Extra pillows or a 'wedge' (you may be able to borrow one of these from your antenatal teacher if you've been to private classes), or birthing stool – a special kidney-shaped stool which some women find it helpful to squat on during labour – if you'd like to try one

What to pack in your suitcase

For yourself
- 3–4 nursing bras
- 2–3 front-opening cotton or cotton-mix nighties
- Plenty of pairs of knickers to hold towels in place
- Paper tissues

PREGNANCY

- Super-absorbent sanitary towels
- Toilet bag containing soap, flannel, brush and comb
- Make-up, shampoo, mousse, mirror
- Breast cream or ointment
- Photo of your husband, other children, pets, etc.
- Coins for phone
- Birth announcement cards and stamps
- Magazines, books, crosswords, notebook and pencil, letter-writing gear, and so on
- Loose outfit to wear for going home

For the baby
- Nappies
- Baby lotion and cotton wool, or baby wipes
- Set of clothes for going home in, consisting of vest, stretch suit, carrying shawl, hat, mitts

WHAT TO BUY FOR YOUR BABY

Buying clothes and equipment for your expected baby is one of the most pleasant tasks during pregnancy. You don't need to buy masses of new things, as you'll almost certainly be given plenty and new babies grow very fast.

Just what and how much you'll need depends on the time of year you are expecting your baby – winter arrivals obviously need more than summer ones – and on your washing and drying facilities. Baby clothes don't get much wear while your baby is still immobile, but you'll need several changes for the inevitable occasions when his nappy leaks or he brings up part of his feed.

Clothes
- 4–6 wide-necked cotton vests
- 4–6 all-in-one towelling or velour stretch suits
- 2–3 cardigans or matinee jackets
- All-in-one padded pram suit, or hat, jacket, mitts and leggings
- Sun hat and parasol for a summer baby

- Carrying shawl or cotton cellular blanket, 'cocoon' or sleeping bag
- 2 pairs socks, bootees and mittens for a winter baby

Changing and bathing

- 20–30 best quality towelling nappies if you're planning to use them *or*
- 10 packs of first-size disposable nappies
- 6 pairs of small waterproof pants (you may find the tie-on ones create a snugger fit in the early days)
- Packet of nappy liners – preferably one way, to keep his bottom dry between changes
- Packet of safety pins
- Changing mat (optional but convenient)
- Large pack of cotton wool
- Tissues
- Baby lotion
- Packet of baby wipes (useful for when you are going out, to save carrying nappy-changing equipment with you)
- Mild baby soap or all-in-one bath solution
- Large soft towel
- Pair of blunt-ended scissors
- Baby hairbrush
- Sponge or two flannels
- Moulded plastic baby bath and stand (optional – you can just as easily bath your baby in the sink, washbasin or a large washing-up bowl)

Bedding

- 2 fitted waterproof sheets
- 3 fitted cotton sheets
- 1 cot-sized duvet and two covers *or*
- 3 top sheets and 3 cellular blankets and an eiderdown
Set of the same in pram/crib size

Feeding

Breast-feeding

- 3 adjustable nursing bras in cotton or cotton-mix
- 1 packet breast pads (not plastic backed)
- Hand breast pump (optional)
- 1 tube of nipple cream or plain lanolin

You may also like to buy a couple of bottles and teats for giving drinks of water or, later on, juice.

Bottle-feeding (see pages 170–73)
- 6–8 wide-necked bottles with teats and covers
- Large graduated measuring jug
- Knife or spatula
- Tins of modified baby milk suitable for a newborn baby
- Sterilizing unit, or covered plastic container such as large freezer carton
- Sterilizing fluid or tablets
- Bottle brush

Buying baby clothes

- Avoid buying too many first-size clothes.
- Choose clothes that are easy to put on and take off – the time for high-fashion garments, if you want them, is later, not when your baby is as slippery as an eel.
- Don't buy too much – you will probably be given lots of presents.
- Avoid fiddly fastenings and anything open-weave that could trap your baby's fingers.
- Go for soft, comfortable fabrics – cotton is best, as some babies are allergic to synthetics or wool.
- Check washing instructions and avoid garments that need to be hand-washed.

Choosing a cot

- Make sure the bars have spaces no more than 3–6 cm (1¼–2½ in.) between them, so your baby cannot get his head stuck through them.
- Check that castors are lockable.
- Check drop-sides to ensure they have a safety-catch and that the baby's fingers cannot get trapped in them.
- Choose a firm, well-ventilated mattress.
- Make sure the cot is firm and stable and that it can't be tipped.
- Look for BSI number 1753 which shows that the cot conforms to strict safety standards set by the British Standards Institute.

Cots

The type of cot you buy for your baby will depend on your pocket and how long he is going to sleep there. A crib or Moses basket looks pretty, and your baby may feel comfortably snug in something this size during the early weeks. However, it isn't essential as he will quickly grow out of it, and you can equally well let him sleep in his carrycot or even a well-padded cupboard drawer.

A drop-sided cot will seem to swamp him at first but you can always place him in it in his carrycot until he's a little older. A cot with an adjustable base and removable sides will last your baby for several years; you can pad the ends and sides to make him feel more secure.

Prams and pushchairs

What you choose will depend both on your purse and your lifestyle. If you don't have access to a car, do your shopping by foot and plan to have another baby fairly soon, you may find the coach-built type most suitable, as it is sturdy, safe for your baby, has plenty of space for shopping and is capable of taking a toddler seat.

Alternatively, if you travel frequently by car, live in a flat where space is at a premium, or need something that is easily collapsible for taking on public transport, then one of the buggy-style prams that converts into a pushchair will be more useful.

Choosing a pram or pushchair

- Check that it has a strong, easy-to-reach brake, and that it is stable and cannot be tipped over.
- Look for space to fit a shopping tray – this is safer than hanging shopping bags over a handle.
- Check that there are anchor points for a safety harness.
- Choose a model that feels comfortable to push and manoeuvre.
- If buying a folding model check that there is a safety device to prevent it collapsing.
- Check for loose parts.
- Look on the label for BSI numbers 4139 for a pram and 4792 for a pushchair which show that they meet safety requirements set by the British Standards Institute.

PREPARING YOUR BABY'S ROOM

Your baby doesn't need a fully furnished room of his own right from the start, although, obviously, if you have space to make him a nursery you may like to do so. He can just as easily have a space in your room or part of another room.

There's no need to spend a lot of money decorating and equipping the room, as your baby will soon outgrow his early needs. Your baby's requirements in the early days are simple, and you may be able to convert or adapt existing furniture or pick up pieces from a second-hand shop. He will need:

- A cot, crib or carrycot (see above).
- A sturdy surface, such as the top of a chest of drawers or table, on which to change his nappy.
- An adjustable light for night feeds and changing.
- A shelf or drawer for storing toiletries.
- A small cupboard, wardrobe or chest of drawers in which to keep his clothes.
- An oil-filled radiator or other safe heater for back-up heating if the weather gets chilly.

FURNISHING THE NURSERY

Make sure all surfaces are clean and easy to wipe down. Carpet tiles, vinyl or cork tiles are easy to clean and convenient for the floor; avoid loose mats, which you could slip on. Decorate the room with bright, cheerful colours, using a non-toxic, lead-free paint. Babies love bright primaries and bold patterns.

Have a table and a low armchair in the room, which are handy for feeding, and fit a dimmer switch to the existing light fitting, convenient for night feeds.

YOUR FEELINGS DURING PREGNANCY

Pregnancy is a time of upheaval in all areas of your life. Not only is your body undergoing dramatic changes but your whole way of life is about to change too. It's hardly surprising that your emotions may be erratic, especially during the first and last three months of pregnancy.

On some days you may feel wildly excited and happy, on others you may feel moody and depressed. You may wonder how you will ever cope with all the new responsibilities. You may worry about your baby's well-being and have vivid dreams or nightmares involving birth and babies. Towards the end of your pregnancy, although you are restless and tired and longing for your baby to be born, you may also feel that you are not ready for the impending birth and wish that you could cancel the whole thing! It's a rare pregnant woman who hasn't felt some or all of these conflicting emotions.

It helps to talk about how you are feeling, to your husband or to a close relative or friend. You may feel especially drawn to your mother or other women who are pregnant at this time. One of the good reasons for attending antenatal classes is that you meet other women who are undergoing the same experiences and can share your confusion and anticipation. Strong bonds are often made between women attending these classes. Many continue to meet and offer vital support to each other after their babies are born.

It is natural to feel anxious too. Most babies are born normal, but the strong fears you feel may be nature's way of helping you mentally prepare in the unlikely event that your baby is ill or handicapped. If anxiety is getting out of hand, causing you severe problems in sleeping, or if you regularly get uncontrollable panic attacks, then do consult your doctor or midwife. You can be helped.

YOU AND YOUR HUSBAND

During pregnancy all the attention tends to be focused on you. The fact that you are to become a mother is immediately evident by your bump. Although your husband has no physical evidence of his impending parenthood, far-reaching changes are about to take place in his life too. He may worry about you and the baby, and may fear for your safety during the birth. He may be concerned about his ability both to cope as a father and, if you are giving up work, to provide for his new family. If there are worries over work, money or housing, all these can add to the

---

Tips to stay close

- Make the most of these last precious months together.
- Share pursuits that you both enjoy, such as going for walks, eating out at restaurants, visiting the theatre or cinema, and so on.
- Prepare for the birth of your baby together. Your husband will be invited to one of the NHS antenatal classes, or you may prefer to seek out a course of classes you can both attend (see page 76).
- If one of you needs time out for a new pursuit, try to allow this space without feeling left out or resentful.
- Share your feelings with each other.
- Don't let misunderstandings fester.

burden of anxiety. Some men feel pushed out by their partner's pregnancy.

Some men faced with their wife's pregnancy feel the need to throw themselves into a new hobby or sport, or to work overtime. It's essential to confide your feelings and worries in each other, and to make a real effort to understand how you are each feeling.

YOUR OTHER CHILDREN

Most parents worry that older children may feel jealous or pushed out by a new arrival. Recent research shows that although temporary upsets are common around the time of the birth, most of these problems will have disappeared by the time the baby is eight months old. No connection has been established between these upsets and the chance of establishing a happy brother/sister relationship.

If you have other children you will have to tell them about the impending arrival. How and when depends on their ages, stages of development and personality. A pre-school child has a short memory and will not be able to understand if you tell her in the first few months before the pregnancy is visible. Be guided by your child's natural curiosity as to when to introduce the subject of your pregnancy. Wait until questions about the growing size of your tummy arise to introduce her gradually to the idea. Older school-age children can be told earlier on in pregnancy and may enjoy watching a video or looking at a book with you outlining the changes in your body. Again be guided by your knowledge of your child to decide when to introduce the idea. Don't overwhelm her with too much information all at once. Give her time to assimilate what you tell her.

Involve your other children in the pregnancy in a way that is suitable to their ages and stage of development. A two- to-three-year-old may like to accompany you when you go for a routine antenatal visit and listen to the baby's heart through the midwife's stethoscope. Plan to take her for a visit that you know will involve just the routine checks, as she will be bored if she has to wait around and you are likely to be less relaxed as a result.

How your child will react when the baby is born will depend on her age and personality, and also, studies suggest, on her relationship with her parents before the birth of the new arrival. Children over the age of five are the least likely to appear upset. Pre-school children may go through a phase of increased naughtiness, clinging or withdrawn behaviour. A toddler who has recently been potty trained frequently goes back to wetting her nappies for a while, and sleep disturbances are also common.

Aim to make any major changes in your child's life, such as transferring her to a big bed, starting playgroup or nursery, and so on, well before the baby's arrival, so that she doesn't feel that she is being pushed out. Alternatively wait until a few months after the baby's birth.

Involve your child in preparing for the baby. She may like to help you prepare the crib or cot, and you can buy a present for her to give the baby. Don't forget to get a little present 'from the baby' for her too.

Make sure she is familiar with the person who is going to look after her while you have the baby. Rehearse what will happen to you with a doll or teddy: 'going to hospital' games will help familiarize her with what will happen and give her the opportunity to work out any worries she may have.

You can minimize the chances of problems occurring by applying a mixture of common sense and tact. It makes sense not to be holding the baby when your older child visits for the first time. You can tell her about the birth of the baby, and let her natural curiosity do the rest. She may like to touch the baby gently, and exchange any presents you have organized on this occasion.

Once you have returned home try to mete out plenty of attention to your older child. Talk to her about the baby as a person, and encourage her to help and become involved in caring for the baby. Problems most often occur when you are bathing, cuddling or feeding the baby. Try to forestall demands for attention by collecting plenty of things to occupy your older child, such as books, crayons, puzzles, plus anything she might need such as the potty or a drink, before carrying out these tasks.

YOUR SEX LIFE

You may wonder what happens to your sex life once you are pregnant. So long as your pregnancy is normal there's no reason why you shouldn't continue to enjoy sex right through pregnancy. Making love is a wonderful way to stay close and cement the bond between you. Many couples find a new enjoyment in sex during pregnancy.

However, there may be a few complications. For instance, some women find their sex drive increases during pregnancy; others experience diminished desire. Many fathers-to-be find the pregnant body uniquely beautiful, but a few can't come to terms with their partner's blossoming shape or they may worry about injuring the baby during love-making. If either of you have other fears or anxieties these, too, can interfere with your desire to make love. All these reactions are normal and understandable.

Problems can occur if one of you wants to make love and the other doesn't. If this happens it is important not to let the matter become a bone of contention between you. Talk over your feelings and reassure each other that they don't arise from any lack of love. Even if you don't find the idea of intercourse appealing, there are many forms of love play you can practise to give each other the excitement, warmth and security you both need. Massage, oral sex, and kissing and cuddling are all good ways of expressing your love and affection.

If you both feel like making love it's perfectly safe to do so as much as you want. In the later stages of pregnancy you may find deep thrusting uncomfortable, so ask your partner to go easy – slow, steady thrusts may be more comfortable and enjoyable. As your bump gets bigger you may feel squashed in positions where your husband is on top. Go for positions in which you are on top, side by side, or any position in which your partner enters you from behind.

Towards the end of pregnancy you may find that a strong climax sets off a string of the painless practice contractions known as Braxton-Hicks. These are not at all harmful and cannot cause you to go into labour prematurely. If you are ready to give birth to your baby they may continue and develop into the true contractions of labour proper.

If you've had a threatened miscarriage your doctor may advise you to abstain from making love for a while. The advice does not, however, imply that intercourse provoked the bleeding – it is given simply as a precautionary measure.

RIGHTS AND BENEFITS AT WORK

If you enjoy your work and are fit and well during pregnancy there is no reason why (with the exceptions outlined below) you shouldn't continue to work. The conventional time to give up your job is around the 28th week of pregnancy, but so long as you remain healthy it is not always necessary to give up then. If in doubt ask the advice of your doctor. Working helps keep you busy and interested, gives you the companionship of your colleagues, and helps stop you dwelling on some of the more uncomfortable aspects of pregnancy, such as morning sickness, as well as providing you with an income at a time when you may well find your financial resources stretched more than usual. Of course, you shouldn't overdo things, and there are some important health factors to bear in mind.

Health hazards

There are a few tasks that you shouldn't do when you are pregnant. If your work involves any of the following you would be advised to stop work or seek an alternative for the duration of your pregnancy:

- Strenuous or dangerous manual work, or work that involves lifting heavy weights.
- Jobs that expose you to excessive noise, heat, or stress.
- Jobs that bring you into contact with poisonous chemicals such as lead, mercury, anaesthetic gases.
- Jobs that involve contact with high levels of radiation.
- Jobs that bring you into contact with potentially harmful infections.
- Jobs that involve working long shifts, periods standing up or excessive amounts of travel.

If you have a previous history of miscarriage, bleeding during pregnancy or premature labour you should also stop work.

VDUs and photocopiers

Visual display units and photocopiers both involve low levels of radiation. There has been no conclusive evidence, despite many studies, that these are harmful to the unborn baby. However, to reduce any possible risk you could ask to be transferred to a machine with no risk of radiation if possible, and stand well back from the machine when making a photocopy. VDUs can cause eyestrain, and sitting in one position for a long time can be uncomfortable when you are pregnant. If you work with one, aim to take regular breaks. If you are worried at all contact your trade union representative or personnel officer for further advice.

Practicalities

When you decide to tell people at work that you are pregnant will depend on a number of factors. If your work is hazardous to pregnant women (see above), or if nausea is interfering with your work then you may want to break the news as soon as your pregnancy is confirmed. However, there is much to be said for delaying revealing your pregnancy until after the first few months are past. Some women prefer to wait until the risk of miscarriage or of termination for abnormality is over.

Although you can carry on working quite happily during pregnancy, you can't ignore the fact that you are pregnant, and would be unwise to do so. A few sensible measures will help you enjoy being pregnant at work:

- If you suffer from morning sickness, pack a selection of snack foods to nibble during the day. Eat little and often. For other tips on coping with morning sickness see page 84.
- Make sure you get enough sleep. Go to bed earlier on working days, and use the weekends for rest and relaxation rather than rushing around.
- Get some rest during the day. If you are lucky enough to have a rest room at work, spend ten minutes with your feet up during the lunch hour. Otherwise try to find a quiet corner or nearby park or open space where you can relax for a short time.
- Rest when you get home from work. Allow yourself half an hour to recover before embarking on any chores – or better still, get your husband to do them.
- Pay attention to your posture at work. Take in a foot stool, or rest your feet on a pile of books. Place a cushion in the small of your back. Get up and walk around at regular intervals.
- Wear support tights and low-heeled shoes for comfort. Some offices get very hot. Wear light layers that you can strip off if it gets stuffy.
- If you can afford it, invest in some help in the home.
- Cut down on your social life if it causes you extra stress.
- Streamline travel arrangements. It may be possible to arrange to work flexible hours so as to avoid the rush hour. You may find it more convenient to change your mode of transport, for example change from train to bus if a bus route passes close to your home. You may be able to drive in to work, or get a lift. If you do travel on public transport don't be afraid to ask politely for someone to give up their seat if it is not offered.
- Eat healthily. It may be better to take in a home-prepared lunch if the local sandwich bar only serves greasy snacks.

As a mother-to-be you have four basic rights at work:

1. Paid time off to visit the antenatal clinic.
2. The right not to be dismissed, unless your job is unsuitable for a pregnant woman. In this case, your boss should offer you another job, if one is available, for the duration of your pregnancy.
3. The right to go back to work after you have had your baby (see below).
4. The right to Statutory Maternity Pay (see below).

In order to qualify for the last two rights, you must:

- Have worked for two years for your employer full-time (i.e. 16 hours or more a week).
- Have worked for five years for your employer part-time (i.e. 8–16 hours a week).

However, you won't be able to go back to work if your job is redundant, if it is impractical for you to return to your job and there is no other suitable position available; or if your firm employs fewer than six people and it is not reasonably practical for you to go back.

Letters to your employer

In order to keep your job open you must write to your employer.

Letter one (written three weeks before you leave work)
Dear Mr/Ms X,
    I am leaving work to have a baby, which is expected on . . . After my baby is born I intend to return to work.

Letter two (reply to the letter your employer may write to you seven weeks after your baby is born, asking you if you still wish to return)
Dear Mr/Ms X,
    Thank you for your letter of . . . I write to confirm that I still intend to come back to work.

Letter three (written at least three weeks before you go back to work)
Dear Mr/Ms X,
    I write to let you know that I will be returning to work on . . .

PREGNANCY

CLAIMING YOUR RIGHTS

Right	How to claim
1. Paid time off for maternity care	Ask your boss for time off. After your first antenatal, show him or her the certificate (Mat B1) that confirms your pregnancy.
2. The right not to be dismissed	If you are dismissed because of pregnancy complain to an industrial tribunal. If you have been fairly dismissed (for instance, because your employer had no alternative suitable work for you during pregnancy) you may still have the right to return to your former job. Check with the Department of Employment.
3. The right to return to work	a. Continue to work until the 11th week before your baby is due (i.e. week 29). b. Give your employer three weeks' notice in writing of your intention to return. c. Show your boss your maternity certificate (Mat B1). d. Tell your employer and confirm in writing that you are returning to work at least three weeks before you do so. e. Return to work before the end of the 29th week after your baby's birth.
4. The right to Statutory Maternity Pay	a. Give your employer at least three weeks' notice of the date you are leaving to have your baby. b. Produce your maternity certificate (Mat B1) within three weeks of your leaving date.

STATUTORY MATERNITY PAY

This is paid by your employer who claims it back from the government.

You are entitled to it whether or not you intend to return to work. In order to qualify:

- You must have worked for your employer without a break except for sickness for six months by the time you are six months (26 weeks) pregnant (i.e. 15 weeks before your baby is due).
- Your average wage (including overtime and bonuses) must have been enough for you to be eligible to pay National Insurance during the 19th to 26th weeks of your pregnancy.
- You must carry on working for your employer until you are 26 weeks pregnant.

If your baby is born early or if you were dismissed before the 26th week of your pregnancy you may still be able to claim SMP. If you aren't eligible for SMP you may be able to claim Maternity Allowance (see below).

When do I receive SMP?

SMP is payable for up to 18 weeks. There is a 'core period' of 13 weeks, which starts six weeks before your baby's estimated date of delivery (EDD). You can claim the other five weeks' pay either before or after the 'core period', or opt to receive some before and some after. SMP is not paid for any week or part week in which you work.

How much do I receive?

There are two rates of SMP, both of which are subject to income tax and National Insurance:

1. *Higher rate* This is 90 per cent of your normal average wage. You receive it for the first six weeks of the 'core period', provided that:

- You have worked for two years for the same employer full-time.
- You have worked for five years for the same employer part-time.

After the period of six weeks you receive the lower rate for the remaining 12 weeks.

2. *Lower rate* This is a set flat rate. For the current rate consult the DSS. You receive it if you've worked at the same job for between 26 weeks and two years.

RIGHTS AND BENEFITS — WHAT TO DO WHEN

When	What you must do
As soon as pregnancy is confirmed	1. Ask your doctor or midwife for form FW8. 2. See your dentist. 3. Read leaflets MV11, H11 and G11 available from the DSS. 4. Tell your employer you are pregnant. 5. Find out whether you are eligible for Maternity Allowance.
Three weeks before giving up work	Write to your employer.
After six months of pregnancy	1. Obtain your maternity certificate (Mat B1) from your doctor or midwife. 2. Give form Mat B1 to your employer. 3. Obtain form MA1 from the DSS or antenatal clinic if you are ineligible for SMP.
After seventh month	1. Apply for Social Fund Maternity Payment if you are eligible. 2. Find out whether you can claim SMP or Maternity Allowance.
After 34 weeks	1. Stop work by the end of this week in order to be eligible for full SMP or Maternity Allowance.
As soon as you can after your baby is born	1. Register the baby's birth. 2. Send off application form for Child Benefit and One Parent Benefit (if you are eligible). 3. Find out whether you are eligible for any other low income benefits.
By six weeks after birth (three weeks in Scotland)	Register the baby's birth.
Seven weeks after EDD	Reply to letter from your employer.
Three weeks before you go back to work	Write to your employer.
Three months after birth	Apply for Maternity Payment if you are eligible.
Before the end of the 29th week after your baby's birth	Return to work.

Why

1. So that you can apply for free prescriptions.
2. To apply for free treatment.
3. To check your rights to benefits.

4. To check whether you are eligible for SMP and to make sure you have time off to keep your antenatal appointments.
5. If you are not eligible for SMP you may be eligible for this allowance.

To protect your rights to SMP and to return to work.

1. To claim SMP or Maternity Allowance.

2. To protect your right to SMP and enable your employer to calculate the allowance to which you are entitled.
3. To claim Maternity Allowance.

1. To buy clothes and equipment for your baby.

2. Payments can begin from now.

1. If you work after this week you may not be entitled to the full sum.

1. To get the baby's birth certificate and NHS card.
2. and 3. To claim these benefits.

Latest date for registration.

To protect your right to return to work.

To protect your right to return to work and to confirm the return date.

You will lose your claim if you don't apply by now.

Failure to do so by this date, except in special circumstances, such as illness, may lose you the right to return.

MATERNITY ALLOWANCE

If you are ineligible for SMP because you are self-employed or have given up work or changed jobs too early to qualify you may be entitled to Maternity Allowance, which is paid by the DSS. In order to qualify you must have worked and paid National Insurance for at least six months of the year that ends when you are six months pregnant.

When do I receive it?
You receive payment for 18 weeks, starting 11 weeks before your baby's EDD. The 'core period' is the same as for SMP but there is only one, flat rate allowance.

How do I claim?
Fill in form MA1, which is available from your local Social Security Office, Citizen's Advice Bureau, Health Centre or antenatal clinic.

SOCIAL FUND MATERNITY PAYMENT

If you or your husband are on Income Support or Family Credit and if your savings are less than a certain amount you can claim a lump sum payment to help defray the cost of maternity clothes and baby equipment. Consult your local DSS for details.

How do I claim?
Write to or call into your local Social Security Office and ask for a claim form. You'll need to take along your Maternity Certificate (Mat B1) or your antenatal clinic card. You should claim as soon as you are 29 weeks pregnant, up until three months after your baby is born. Don't delay claiming or you may lose your payment.

OTHER BENEFITS

As a pregnant woman you are also eligible for:

- Free prescriptions
- Free dental treatment
- Free milk and vitamins if you are on Income Support.

How do I claim?
Once your pregnancy is confirmed fill in form FW8, which is available from your doctor or midwife.

Part II

LABOUR AND BIRTH

Presentation

The way your baby lies in the womb is called the presentation. Towards the end of pregnancy your baby settles into position ready to be born. There are many different ways to give birth. Some of these have been outlined in the section dealing with birth choices (pages 41–2). Other factors that will affect the type of birth you have are your own and the baby's health, and the way your baby is lying in the uterus (see below). You will feel more relaxed and comfortable if you know what to expect during labour and if you have become familiar with ways to help yourself. If you have been to classes, you may be familiar with the layout of the labour ward, and may even have met some of the team who will be caring for you. If you are giving birth at home, you will have made all your preparations, and can relax and enjoy the birth.

Your baby's head is the largest, heaviest part of him, and for this reason most babies take up the traditional head-down, or cephalic, position before birth. In fact, 95 per cent of babies are lying head down by the 37th week of pregnancy. During birth the baby's head rotates down through the birth canal.

The ideal position for a natural, normal birth is with the baby's head down and the back against your abdomen. This way, your baby has less distance to rotate in the birth canal, and the narrowest part of his head will be the first to enter it. When your baby lies in this way it is called the occipito anterior position.

More unusual is the occipito posterior position, in which the baby's head is down but his back is towards your spine. This tends to make for a longer labour, especially of the second stage, since the baby has further to rotate in the birth canal. Occasionally a baby does not make the turn and is born looking up at you.

About 3–4 per cent of babies stay in the breech position, that is, with bottom down and head up. Some babies turn around even after the 37th week of pregnancy, but in most cases if your baby hasn't turned by this date you can expect a breech delivery (see page 150) or even a caesarean (see page 147).

If you go into labour with your baby in the breech position the hospital staff will want to keep a particularly careful eye on your progress. The problem with a breech is that the baby's head, which is

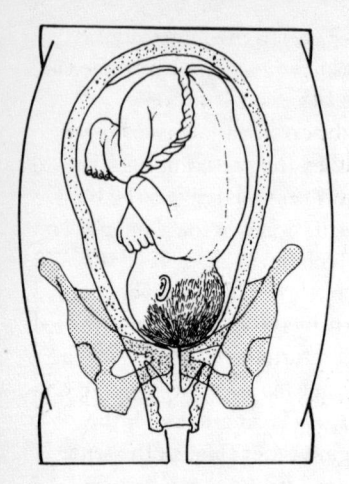

LABOUR AND BIRTH

Occipito anterior position

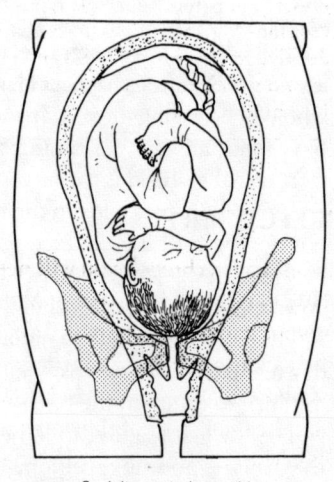

Occipito posterior position

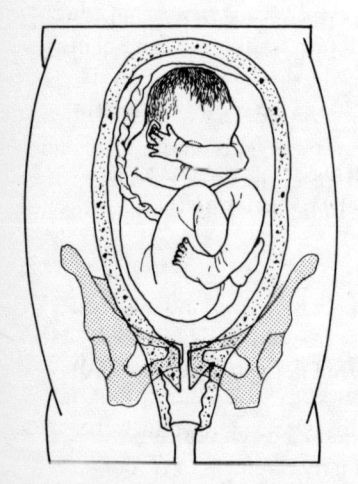

Breech position

the largest part of the body, is delivered last, when the birth canal is not sufficiently well stretched. For this reason you will probably need an episiotomy and forceps delivery (see pages 145 and 146). Some obstetricians prefer to deliver all breeches by caesarean to avoid injury to the baby's head, while others claim that if you can stay upright to give birth it is possible to achieve an entirely normal delivery.

To turn a breech baby

If your baby is still breech by 37 weeks you may like to encourage him to turn yourself. Lie on your back on the floor and place a cushion or two under your pelvis. Stay in this position, with your bottom raised on the cushions, for 15 minutes or so, two or three times a day. Relax and breathe deeply, and move your hips gently up and down from time to time. If you feel your baby turn stay upright for an hour or two to give him time to settle into his new position.

BREECH BIRTH

If your baby is breech you will need to have a hospital birth. Just before delivery you will be given an X-ray to ensure that there is enough room for your baby's head to pass through your pelvis. You'll also be scanned to check the baby's proportions.

Labour may be longer and slower than usual because the head, which is the heaviest part of the body, comes out last, unlike in a normal birth when the gravity of the baby's head assists the opening of the cervix. Keeping upright and moving around will help labour progress faster.

Transverse position Very rarely a baby is lying across the uterus, in which case a caesarean section is almost always performed.

TWINS

If there is a history of twins in your family, or if you seem to be much larger than your dates suggest, you may suspect you are carrying twins. The minor discomforts and aches and pains of pregnancy tend to be exaggerated when you are having twins.

Confirmation is by your first ultrasound scan, usually at around 16 weeks, or by the midwife picking up two heart beats during her examination at an antenatal. By the time your babies are large enough to be palpated the doctor or midwife will usually be able to detect two bodies when feeling your abdomen, although occasionally one baby may be lying directly behind the other. In the past this was one reason why twins sometimes went undetected until birth. Today with the advent of ultrasound this event is virtually unheard of.

Tips to help you cope with a twin pregnancy

- Make time for extra rest and relaxation.
- Get as much help as you can. If you have other children, try to find someone who will take them off your hands from time to time, to allow you to rest. If you are still working try to put your feet up in the lunch hour.
- Go swimming – it is a good all-round exercise and has the added advantage of taking the weight off your bump.
- Take special care over your diet, as the babies will make extra demands on your resources.
- Invest in some pretty maternity outfits, as you'll need to go into pregnancy clothes at an earlier stage than mothers of single babies.
- Beg or borrow as many cast-offs as you can to make up your babies' layette. It may be easier to use disposable nappies, even though this is obviously expensive.
- Cut housework to the minimum and try to get help in the home. Ask your midwife if you are eligible for a home help.
- Make practical arrangements well in advance for having other children looked after while you are in hospital, packing your bag, and so on, in case your twins are born early.

Coping with a twin pregnancy

You may find that the tiredness, nausea, varicose veins, and so on, of normal pregnancy are much more marked when you are expecting twins. For many mothers-to-be, the excitement and anticipation of planning for two babies help make these discomforts more bearable. However, if the twins have come as a shock, you may need a little while to come to terms with the idea. Talk to your husband, and your midwife and, through the Twins and Multiple Births Association, contact a mother who already has twins to see how she copes (see page 204 for address).

Twin pregnancies are usually shorter than for a single baby. The doctor will want to monitor you particularly carefully, and you may be advised to attend extra antenatal checks. Certainly you should have your babies in hospital, as there is a greater chance of complications arising during labour. A twin pregnancy places increased demands on your body, so it's especially important to look after yourself. Particular attention will be paid to your weight gain, and blood pressure to ensure that you are not developing pre-eclampsia.

Twin presentation

Identical twins usually share the same placenta; most non-identical twins have separate placentas. There are three main types of twin presentation:

1. Both twins lying head down (cephalic): about 50 per cent of twins lie this way.
2. One twin head down, the other breech: a common twin presentation. The head-down twin is usually born first. Forceps will probably be needed for the second twin but, as the birth canal will already have been stretched by the first twin, delivery is usually straightforward.
3. Both twins are breech: this is more unusual and your twins will probably be delivered by caesarean section.

Engagement of the head or 'lightening'

At around 36 to 38 weeks if you are expecting your first baby, but often not until you go into labour with second and subsequent babies, your baby's head settles deep down in your pelvis, or engages. When this happens you'll feel a relief of pressure in your abdomen, which is why it is sometimes called 'lightening', and breathing will be easier as your baby is no longer pressing up against your diaphragm and lungs.

POSITIONS FOR LABOUR

First stage

Staying upright and remaining active can help you feel more comfortable.

1. Lean against a wall, your husband or your labour companion while you have a contraction. As you do so he or she can massage your lower back to give you relief.

LABOUR AND BIRTH

2. Kneel down and lean your head against your arms, using a chair with a cushion on it for support. Between contractions rest to one side.
3. If you are becoming tired, try kneeling on all fours. Rock backwards and forwards and rotate your pelvis. Rest back on your heels to one side between contractions.
4. Sit on a chair facing its back and rest your head on your arms against the back of the chair. Use a cushion for comfort.
5. Squat leaning forward on to your hands for support and rock your weight from hands to feet. If your arms ache shake or massage them, or get your husband to, between contractions.
6. Sit on the edge of the bed, feet up on a couple of stools for comfort, leaning against your husband. If you like he can massage your back or thighs.

Second stage

1. Stand with your husband and the midwife or helper on either side of you and put your arms around their shoulders, then squat while fully supported. You can do this on a bed or on a mattress on the floor.
2. Stand with your husband behind you supporting you under the armpits. When you feel the urge to push relax your knees as he takes your weight.
3. Kneel on the bed with husband and helper for support.
4. If you prefer to lie back, prop yourself into as upright a position as you can, using pillows or cushions for support. Your partner can sit behind you and hold you if you like.

Tips for travelling to hospital

- If you're travelling to hospital by car make sure you have a full tank of petrol.
- Make a few trial runs in different traffic conditions between home and hospital so you can estimate the length of the journey.
- If you're planning to go to hospital by ambulance check the instructions on the front of your co-operation card.
- If you're planning to go by taxi make sure you have the numbers of several taxi companies by the telephone.
- Make yourself comfortable on the journey with a cushion at the base of your spine. You may be more comfortable travelling in the back seat. Your husband or whoever takes you to hospital should drive steadily and with care, avoiding sudden braking or sharp swerves.

time limit if this happens). And contractions may become regular for a while and then fade away.

If you are unsure whether labour has begun, try timing contractions over the course of an hour, noting the space between each one, and the length of each contraction. Labour is not established until contractions are progressively closer together and lasting longer than 40 seconds from start to finish. A first labour lasts an average of 12 to 14 hours from the onset of *regular* contractions, so there's plenty of time to be sure you are really in labour before rushing to the hospital. Bearing in mind that contractions will last from one to one-and-a-half minutes, with an interval of one to two minutes between each one towards the end of the first stage, will give you a sense of perspective in the early part of labour.

What is labour?

What sparks off labour remains a mystery, but it's thought that the baby produces hormones that instigate the birth process. During labour your cervix, the neck of the womb, which has been thick and snug around

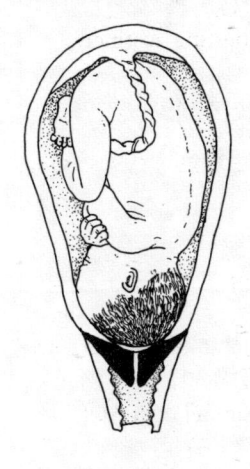

DILATATION OF THE CERVIX

Early labour, the cervix is starting to dilate

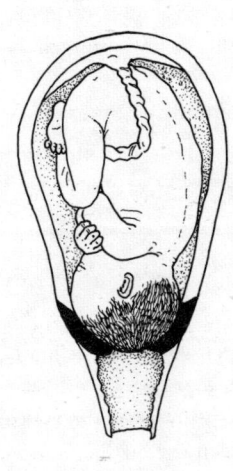

Middle first stage, the cervix continues to widen and be drawn up

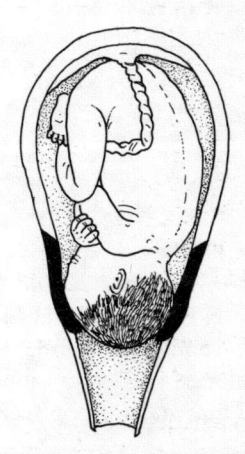

Full dilatation, the cervix is now approximately 10 cm (4 in.) wide at the end of the first stage

LABOUR AND BIRTH

the baby in her protective bag of waters, thins and is drawn up, rather like a polo neck sweater. At the same time, it opens to a width of about 10 cm (4 in.) to allow your baby's head through. When this process – the longest and most uncomfortable part of labour – is complete, your uterus pushes the baby down the birth canal and out into the world. Finally, your baby's lifeline, the placenta, is expelled.

What is a contraction?

A contraction is a regular tightening of the muscles of the uterus. In fact your uterus contracts painlessly at intervals throughout life. During pregnancy your uterus contracts about every 20 minutes, and this ensures good circulation and growth. These slight, painless tightenings are known as Braxton-Hicks contractions (after the doctor who first put a name to them), and you may be totally unaware of them. During the last weeks of pregnancy these contractions begin to prepare the uterus for labour, by drawing up the cervix slightly and making it thinner. Once labour begins, the character of the contractions changes. They become stronger, regular, and more painful. No one knows quite why the contractions of labour are painful. During the first stage of labour the muscle fibres at the top of the uterus contract, producing an upward pull on the cervix so that it is gradually drawn up. As each contraction exerts pressure on the baby's head at the same time the cervix is slowly widened until it forms a continuous birth canal. The contractions of early labour may be irregular and erratic, but gradually they take on a more purposeful character. As they do so you may experience each contraction in the form of a wave-like sensation, which builds up slowly to a crescendo, and then fades away again.

During the second stage of labour the contractions change again producing an irresistible urge to bear down several times during each contraction.

Doctors have conventionally divided labour into three stages:

First stage Your cervix thins and is drawn up ('effaced' is the medical term), and widens (dilates) to form a continuous funnel with your vagina, known as the birth canal.
Second stage Contractions change to the bearing-down variety as the uterus pushes your baby down the birth canal.
Third stage The placenta and bag of membranes is delivered.

In practice, you may experience your labour as a single process. With the increase in epidurals (see page 135), which blur the division between stages, and in natural birth, many obstetricians are beginning to question the rigid time limits previously set and to realize that each labour has a natural tempo of its own. Each labour is different and the ability to adapt your responses to what happens to you is vital.

False labour

In false labour you may think you are in labour, but instead of contractions getting longer, stronger and closer together, they fade away and vanish. There's no need to feel foolish if you think you are in labour but are subsequently proved wrong. Even experts are fooled on occasion. The following pointers may help you decide whether you are truly in labour or not:

- Contractions are short – 10 to 15 seconds.
- Contractions are irregular, or if they do become regular for a while they do not remain so.
- Contractions don't get closer together.
- Contractions often fade if you lie down, whereas in proper labour contractions don't fade when you lie down, though they may be stronger and more effective if you stay upright.

The medical view of labour

The following rule of thumb is often adopted in plotting an individual labour. In practice your labour may be much longer or shorter than these guidelines.

Stages	*First baby*	*Second or subsequent baby*
First stage	12–14 hours	6–10 hours
Second stage	1 hour	30 minutes
Third stage	20–30 minutes	20–30 minutes

How long does labour last?

Doctors who have studied the labours of thousands of women have determined a standard rate at which they believe labour should progress. This is generally accepted as the cervix opening up at a rate of 1 cm (about ½ in.) per hour. If your particular labour diverges from this, the doctor may decide to set up a hormone drip (see page 143) to speed up your labour or 'restore it to normal'.

However, many natural childbirth supporters and midwives point out that each labour has its own natural pace and rhythm: that some women naturally have long, slow labours and that others stop and start.

LABOUR AND BIRTH 124

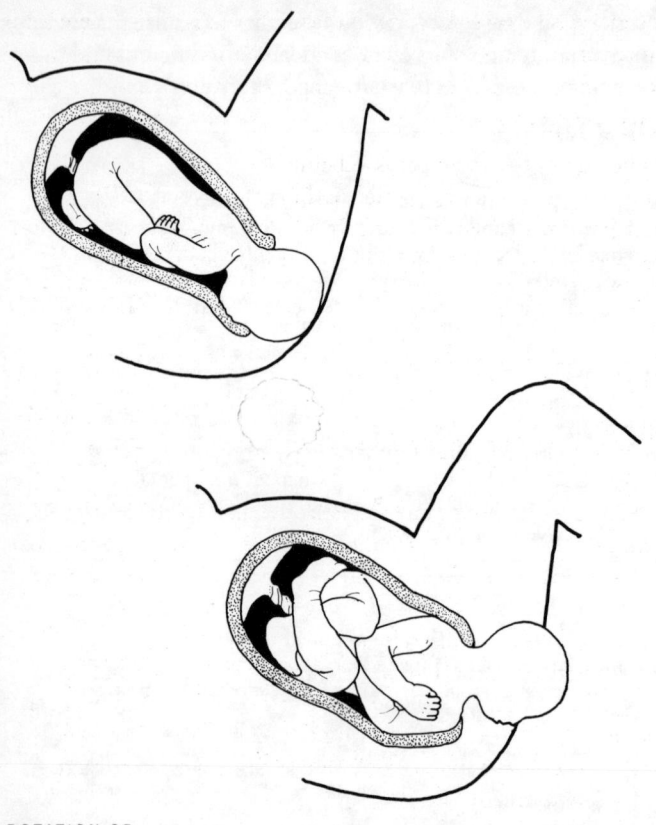

ROTATION OF THE BABY'S HEAD

During the second stage, the baby's head moves down through the pelvis

The head rotates through an angle of 90° and begins to emerge from the birth canal

Once the head is born it rotates again in order to allow the shoulders to lie from front to back – the easiest position in which to ease them out

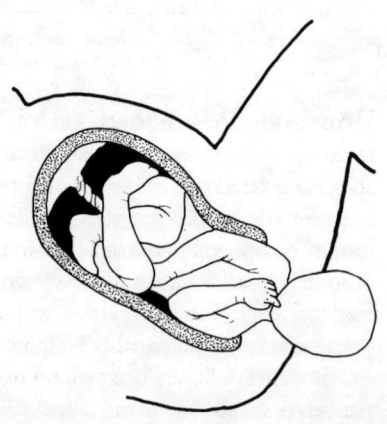

They argue that, so long as labour is measurably progressing, there is no need to interfere.

How will it feel?

Many women describe labour pains as being like very strong period pains – only worse. You may experience the pain in your back – a backache labour – especially if your baby is lying in a posterior position (see page 113). You may get cramp in your thighs or a feeling of stretching low down in your abdomen. Some women experience long, strong contractions right from the start. In others, contractions are irregular in length and strength throughout. Whatever happens contractions become progressively stronger and closer together as you reach the end of the first stage – the most painful part of labour. After this there may be a brief lull before your body begins the work of pushing your baby out.

Second-stage contractions have a quality of their own: the urge to push is completely irresistible. Your job is simply to go along with what your body is telling you to do. You can feel the hardness of your baby's head as it presses between your legs. Some women find this not unpleasant, others say it is like a huge bowel motion.

To start off with, contractions last about 20–30 seconds and occur about every 20 minutes. By the end of the first stage they last between 45 and 60 seconds and occur every two to three minutes. However, you may experience what seems to be one almost continuous contraction, with little space between.

During the second stage, contractions last about 60 to 70 seconds and occur every two to three minutes.

When should I go into hospital?

Labour for a first-time mother lasts on average some 12 to 14 hours, so there's no need to rush to the maternity unit at the first twinge. Labour will seem much shorter and be more bearable if you can ignore it for as long as possible, staying at home in familiar surroundings and pottering around to take your mind off your contractions. You should go into hospital as soon as you feel you would be happier there. The precise point will vary from mother to mother, but most tend to go in too early rather than too late. As a general rule, you may like to go in when contractions are occurring more often than once every five minutes.

Bear in mind that, by the end of the first stage, contractions last one minute and occur every two minutes.

If you've previously had a very fast labour, you may want to go in as soon as you realize you are in labour. There is some controversy as to what you should do if your waters burst. The most usual advice is to go straight away to the hospital. This is because once the cushion of waters that was protecting the baby has gone, the way is open for germs to get into the uterus and cause an infection. The other reason is that sometimes the cord is swept down and compressed by the baby's head, cutting off her supply of oxygen and nutrient-carrying blood. Most doctors prefer to deliver a baby within 12 to 24 hours of the waters bursting to avoid these possibilities. However, sometimes the waters leak a little, and then the bag of waters seals over again. In the case of a leak, you may not even be sure whether your waters have gone or whether it is merely a trickle of urine. In this case it is probably best to carry on as usual unless your baby is more than three weeks early. If your waters go in a gush, you should contact the hospital or your midwife for advice.

Keep a note of the length and frequency of your contractions to give you some idea of the speed at which your labour is progressing.

Ring the hospital before you set off so that they know to expect you and can have your notes and any other relevant information ready for your arrival.

Go to the hospital immediately if:
- You are passing a bright red, heavy flow of blood.
- You have previously had a very fast labour or emergency birth.
- Your baby is coming before 36 weeks.
- Your waters burst.
- Your waters have burst and you are running a temperature (this could be a sign of infection).
- You feel very frightened.
- You feel you would be happier there.

What happens when you reach hospital

When you arrive at the hospital you'll be greeted by a midwife. If you have previously telephoned she will have read your notes and be familiar with your history. You will be taken into a small preparation room or occasionally the room in which you are to spend labour. At this point your husband or labour companion may be asked to wait outside. If you'd like him or her to stay with you, don't be afraid to say so.

The midwife will want to know the time you started having contractions and their frequency, whether you have had a show and whether your waters have broken. She'll time a few contractions to measure their strength and assess how you are coping with them. She'll feel your abdomen to determine the position of the baby. If there is time she will take a urine sample to test for the presence of chemicals called ketones, which could show if you are becoming low on energy, and she'll take your temperature, pulse and blood pressure. She will listen to your baby's heart to find out how she is standing up to labour, by using a fetal stethoscope or, more often nowadays, by putting you on an electronic monitor (see page 128) for a short period. Finally, she will carry out an internal examination to test how far your cervix is dilated. After this she will be able to give you some idea of how your labour is progressing and may even hazard a guess as to the time your baby will be born, although you should remember that this is only an estimate.

Few hospitals now shave off pubic hair, although it may be clipped if it is very long. You may be given an enema or suppository if you haven't had a bowel motion recently, but as mild diarrhoea often precedes labour, chances are you won't need it.

You may be offered a warm bath or shower. (If your waters have broken, it will be a shower to prevent ascending infection.) If your contractions have been painful, you will find that the ache ebbs away in the warmth of the water.

After this you'll be shown to the room where you are to spend either the first stage or, if there is no special delivery room, the rest of your labour. Many labour wards are built on a 'race track' principle, with several single side rooms off corridors around the central nursing station where the staff are based. You'll be allocated a midwife, who may also be looking after one or two other women in labour, and there may be a student midwife present, who may stay with you throughout your labour and who may well deliver your baby. If you are having a Domino delivery, or are giving birth in a GP unit, your midwife may well be the same one who has looked after you during pregnancy and whom you have come to know well. If you are giving birth in a teaching hospital you may be asked if you would be prepared to let a medical student or student nurse view your labour and birth. If you feel you would prefer more privacy you can refuse this request.

MONITORING

Monitoring simply means keeping an eye on you and the baby to make sure you are standing up to the stress and strain of labour. Midwives have always monitored women in labour, using their experience and the skills of hands, eyes and ears to tell how well labour is progressing. Today the word monitoring is more likely to refer to observing by means of electronic machines. The machines are highly sophisticated, and in many maternity units their use has fully complemented the traditional skills of the midwife.

Monitoring refers, in fact, to a set of techniques rather than just one. At its simplest, the midwife uses a hand-held fetal stethoscope to listen to your baby's heart. The length, strength and speed of your baby's heart beat are vital signs, which can warn a skilled midwife or doctor if your baby is running short of oxygen (becoming distressed) and therefore needs to be delivered quickly. The midwife also uses her hands and eyes to observe you and assess the progress of your labour.

Slightly more sophisticated is the Sonicaid, which is carried by many community midwives. A hand-held transducer is passed over your abdomen to pick up and magnify the sound of your baby's heart.

Telemetry is another system, which uses radio waves to pick up your baby's heart rate. Your waters are broken and a scalp electrode is attached to your baby's head. A transducer is strapped around your thigh which passes radio signals to the equipment. Since you are not wired up directly to a piece of machinery, and the radio waves are capable of being carried over some distance, you are able to move around more freely than would be possible with the forms of monitoring described below. Telemetry is not yet widely available.

The cardiotocograph (CTG) is an external electronic monitor that picks up the baby's heart beat and measures the length and strength of your contractions. A belt is strapped around your abdomen, while you lie perfectly still, and is connected to a machine that gives a print-out of your baby's heart rate and shows how it is responding to contractions. This type of monitor may be used when you first go into hospital, and subsequently on and off throughout labour. Towards the end of the first stage of labour, the doctor or midwife may want to monitor you continuously.

If labour is not straightforward an internal monitor may be used. It involves inserting a thin wire through your cervix (your waters will be broken first if they haven't already done so), and attaching a small electrode to the baby's head. A catheter type of transducer is often inserted at the same time to measure contractions. The results of these observations are registered on a print-out in the same way as an external monitor. Internal monitoring is usually extremely accurate, and where problems are suspected it can warn doctors in good time so that the appropriate emergency action may be taken.

The great monitoring debate

No one is denying that monitoring is valuable and can save lives when it is properly used. However, experts disagree on whether electronic monitoring should be used as a routine for all mothers in labour, purely to be on the safe side; or whether it is best reserved for those who need it because their babies are at risk in some way.

Worries have been expressed that electronic monitoring can have a snowball effect, leading to ever more intervention, such as a drip to induce labour, increased need for pain relief and a higher incidence of forceps and caesarean births (see pages 146–7).

External and internal monitors limit free movement, which, say the opponents of monitoring, can lead to a prolonged labour. Occasionally a machine diagnoses a baby as being in distress, and a forceps delivery or even a caesarean is then carried out in order to 'rescue' the baby, who is found to be perfectly healthy at birth. Some studies have shown that electronic monitoring increases the likelihood of such unnecessary intervention. However, with increasingly sophisticated methods of measuring the baby's well-being, such as sampling blood from her scalp or cord, unnecessary operational deliveries may well be avoided.

One valid criticism sometimes raised is that once a machine has been set up, attention may well be concentrated more on the monitor than on the woman on the bed, resulting in a detrimental effect on human relationships during labour. That said, many midwives, trained to use

---

Reasons for monitoring

You will usually be electronically monitored if:

- Labour was induced.
- Labour has been artificially speeded up (accelerated).
- You have had an epidural (see page 135).
- The baby is at high risk, for instance if you have high blood pressure or any other medical condition, or your baby is not growing properly.
- You are expecting twins.

these devices as adjuncts to their traditional skills, often feel happier and more able to attend to the mother's wider needs when a monitor is set up. Many mothers, too, brought up in an age of technology, feel safer knowing they have the back-up of electronic devices.

As always it is important that you are fully informed, so that, with the help and advice of your attendants, you can make realistic choices in whatever situation you find yourself during labour.

A partogram

The course of your labour will be recorded on a special chart called a partogram. The rate at which your cervix is dilating, your baby's heart beat, your blood pressure and pulse are all noted, as well as the appearance of the 'waters', pain relief given, and findings of examinations.

Labour is usually expected to proceed at the rate of 1 cm (½ in.) dilatation per hour. If you fail to progress at this rate the obstetrician may consider accelerating your labour by setting up a hormone drip (see page 143) to strengthen contractions.

PAIN IN LABOUR

How much will it hurt?

There's no doubt that labour is painful, especially towards the end of the first stage. The amount of pain that you feel, however, varies according to the length and strength of your contractions, the way the baby is lying, your individual pain threshold, and so on.

There are several ways of making the pain more bearable. About 50 per cent of women in Britain accept some form of pain relief, but in Holland, where far more births take place at home, there is a lower incidence of drug-use for pain relief. So the way in which you cope relies partly on what you expect and partly on how your attendants try to help you deal with the pain of labour.

Labour pains are different from other sorts of pain in that, although intense, they have a purpose. The knowledge that there is an end to the pain, and that the pains are contributing to the birth of a baby, motivates some women to do without pain relief altogether. And just as a sportsman may not notice an injury in the hurly-burly of the game, so you may be so absorbed in the intensity of labour that you don't feel the need for pain relief. In fact, some research has shown that women who accepted an epidural (see page 135) – the most complete form of pain relief – felt they had missed out on a vital experience.

All the drugs given for pain relief affect the baby in varying degrees and dim your awareness to a certain extent. So, although you should never feel guilty if you accept drugs, you need to weigh up carefully the pros and cons of each method of pain relief, in order to decide on what is best for you.

Pain relief

The type of pain relief you have and the stage at which you accept it will depend on a number of factors both physical and mental. You may need drugs if:

- Labour is very long and contractions are strong.
- You expect labour to be unduly painful.
- You have anticipated that labour will be pain-free, so you are unprepared for the intensity of contractions.
- Your baby is lying in an awkward position.
- You are small and your baby is big.
- Although you have been having contractions, your labour is not progressing.
- You are overtired.
- You are extremely frightened or lonely and therefore your resistance to pain is lowered, partly through tension.

How you can help yourself

There are many ways in which you can help yourself cope with the pain of labour, even if you don't manage to avoid using any form of pain relief altogether. Acknowledging that labour *is* painful can enable you to plan in advance ways in which you might deal with it. Women who have had a drug-free birth often experience a special sense of achievement, although there is no need to feel ashamed if you do accept help.

These are some of the tried-and-tested ways of dealing with pain the drug-free way:

- **Companionship** The company of someone you love and trust – it could be your husband, a friend, relative or even your antenatal teacher – is invaluable. He or she can support and encourage you when you lose heart, can help you make sense of what is happening by pointing out your progress, and can help explain and interpret

your wishes to the staff if you don't feel like doing so for yourself.
- **Movement** Freedom to move around and adopt the most comfortable position for yourself helps ease pain. Staying upright improves blood flow and thus oxygen supply to the uterus and helps it work more efficiently. It's thought that lack of oxygen could be responsible for severe labour pain. Any muscle aches when it is not supplied with enough oxygen. When your uterus is working very hard lack of oxygen may make pain worse (see Breathing below).
- **Food** It is the policy in some units to withhold food and drink from women in labour, on the grounds that there is a danger of regurgitation should an emergency caesarean become necessary. Once you are in established labour you will probably no longer feel like eating anything, although you should still have plenty of drinks and, if you are lacking energy, take spoonfuls of honey or suck glucose sweets. Early on in labour a light, non-greasy snack such as a yoghurt, a slice of bread and honey, a boiled egg, can help keep up your strength. Let your appetite guide you. You probably won't feel like eating anything heavy and, as your labour progresses, your digestive system shuts down and you will cease to feel hungry.
- **Rest** Pain is always more difficult to bear if you are tired. Try to relax completely between contractions. If labour begins at night, try to get some sleep.
- **Warmth** Warmth is enormously soothing – that's the reason a warm shower or bath often makes the pain of contractions ebb away so wonderfully. Feet often get cold in labour, so make sure you have a pair of woolly socks to wear.
- **A home-like atmosphere** Women who give birth at home usually need less in the way of pain relief than those who give birth in hospital. The reason is partly that you feel relaxed in the comfort of your own home. Fortunately, many hospitals are making a real effort to make the labour ward a more homely place. You can enhance the feeling of familiarity by taking along a few things from home – your own nightie, a favourite picture, a vase of flowers.
- **Breathing** At one time complicated breathing routines were taught for use in labour. Perhaps their main value was to distract women from the sensations of labour. At any rate, today it is recognized that, provided you are relaxed, you will breathe in the most appropriate way by instinct. Taking a long, slow breath at the

beginning and end of each contraction will help oxygenate your blood and may relieve pain caused by lack of oxygen to the muscles of the uterus.

- **Positive messages** Your labour companion can help you to think positively by telling you how well you are progressing. You can also buoy yourself up by saying to yourself, 'Now that that contraction has gone, I'm one step nearer to seeing my baby.'
- **Massage** Firm, circular back massage is extremely soothing, especially if you are having a backache labour (see page 136). Some women enjoy light fingertip massage over the abdomen or firm stroking of the thighs. Tell your companion or your midwife what feels best.
- **Distraction or focusing** Some women find they can distract themselves from the pain by chanting a nursery rhyme or simple poem, or focusing on something outside themselves such as a picture or a vase of flowers. Others find such techniques make them feel out of control and prefer to absorb themselves in the experience of labour. Concentrating on your breathing is one good way to do this. It's a technique that is taught in many natural birth classes, and it's probably better to try and learn beforehand. A technique taught in many birth classes involves inhaling deeply through the nose and then breathing out slowly through the mouth, concentrating on this outward breath. Doing this at the start and finish of a contraction can help you to remain calm. It helps to have practised this before you go into labour.

TENS (transcutaneous electrical nerve stimulation) This is a way of helping yourself to cope without forms of pain relief that is becoming increasingly available in hospitals. The method is used widely in Sweden, where about a third of women having babies use it as their only method of pain relief. It works by sending mild electrical charges to the brain, which block the pain sensations and spark off the release of endorphins, the body's own natural pain killers. The TENS equipment consists of a small, hand-held, battery-operated box with electrodes wired up to it. The electrodes are placed on your back at points where some parts of the nerves which serve the cervix and uterus are situated. When the machine is switched on you experience a tingling, prickly sensation that shortly changes to a pleasant, continuous, electrical sensation.

The method doesn't completely eliminate pain – and if you have a long, painful, drawn-out labour, you may need some other form of relief. However, it may delay the time when you need to have pain-relieving drugs and may even, if you are lucky, eliminate their need altogether.

The biggest advantages are that it has no harmful effects on your baby and it enables you to be completely alert and aware.

If you like the idea of using TENS ascertain before you go into hospital to have your baby whether the equipment is available there so you can try it out before you go into labour. If it isn't available you may be able to hire it from a manufacturer (see page 203 for address).

You will probably get the most out of TENS if you start using it early on in labour. Although the conventional placing of the electrodes is on either side of your spine, you may want to experiment to see if you get greater pain relief by applying them to your thighs or even feet.

DRUGS FOR PAIN RELIEF

Pethidine

This is a narcotic (sleep-inducing) drug that has been used widely in labour wards for the last 20 years, although it is currently losing in popularity to the epidural (see page 135). Pethidine can be useful if you are extremely tense, or if there is a 'lip' of cervix which is preventing full dilatation. Sometimes a small rim or lip of cervix is not quite fully taken up even when the rest of the cervix is fully dilated. In this case although you will have a strong urge to push down you may be asked not to do so. Pethidine can sometimes help you to relax until this 'anterior lip', as it is called medically, has disappeared. An alternative is to blow out sharply when you feel a contraction. Kneeling on all fours, with your head down and your bottom up can also help you resist the pushing urge.

It is usually given in the form of an injection into your buttock or thigh, although in some maternity units it may be fed into your wrist via a small pump. The effects vary – it can make you feel pleasantly relaxed and drowsy or dizzy and out of control. It doesn't take away the pain, but it does make you feel slightly distanced from it.

Pethidine starts to work between 10 and 20 minutes after the injection is given, and effects last two to four hours. Sometimes it is mixed with other drugs to enhance its effect or to prevent vomiting.

Perhaps the major disadvantage of pethidine is that it penetrates through to the baby and, especially if the drug is given between four hours and half an hour before delivery, may make her sleepy, unresponsive and less inclined to feed well in the first few days after birth. Fortunately, an antidote (Narcan) can be given to reverse these effects when your baby is born.

The usual dose is 100–200 mg, but if you are unsure about trying it ask for a small dose to see how you cope with it.

Epidural

This can offer almost total pain relief. It involves injecting an anaesthetic drug into the epidural 'space' that lies between your spinal column and the spinal cord, so numbing the nerves that lead to your womb and the surrounding area. If you are given an epidural you lie curled on your side or bent forward on the edge of the bed. You are first given a local anaesthetic, after which you remain absolutely still while the anaesthetist carefully guides the needle into place. Once it is in position, a fine plastic tube is inserted and taped into place through which top-ups of anaesthetic can be given. The needle is then removed. The epidural takes about 20 minutes to work, after which you should be completely free of pain. Further doses of anaesthetic can be given as required. Inserting the epidural is a highly skilled procedure that is carried out by an anaesthetist, though top-ups can be given by a midwife. If you think you would like an epidural check during pregnancy that such a service is offered at your hospital, and whether or not it is available on a 24-hour basis. In some smaller hospitals there may be long delays before an anaesthetist is available. If this seems likely to happen in the hospital in which you have booked it is better not to pin all your hopes on having an epidural. Think about what other methods of pain relief are available and might suit you.

An epidural can be valuable where labour is long and tiring, or where your baby is lying awkwardly. It is usually the anaesthetic of choice if you go into premature labour, as it has fewer effects on the baby than other types of drug. An epidural lowers blood pressure, which is useful if you are suffering pre-eclampsia, and it also enables you to be awake and aware if you are having your baby by caesarean.

The disadvantage of an epidural is that its use tends to make labour longer and more drawn out. This is partly because you are usually confined to bed once the drug has been administered; and partly because the epidural softens the pelvic floor, so the baby takes longer to rotate in the birth canal. The drug can be finely timed to wear off at the second stage of labour, so that you can push the baby out yourself, but even so there is a higher incidence of forceps deliveries where an epidural has been administered.

If you have an epidural you will need to be carefully monitored, as you won't be able to feel the strength of contractions. You won't be able to feel when you want to pass water, either, so a special fine tube (catheter) may be used to empty your bladder. Very occasionally, the epidural accidentally leaks into the space that protects your spinal cord and allows the escape of spinal fluid. This may cause an excruciating headache, which can, however, be effectively treated.

For a completely pain-free birth, or in the case of complications, an epidural can be the ideal form of pain relief.

Backache labour

If your baby is lying in the posterior position, that is, with her back towards your spine, you may experience labour pains in your back, as the hard back of her head presses against the lower part of your spine. Such a labour can be tiring and stressful, as it is likely to last longer than usual.

- Keep up your strength by having rest and relaxation during the early part of labour.
- Take a walk to help you exercise and relax, and to take your mind off a long, slow labour.
- Keep upright and move around as feels comfortable.
- Apply a hot-water bottle to your lower back, to help soothe pain.
- Exert firm pressure using the heel of the hand on either side of your buttocks, to relieve discomfort; or ask your husband to roll a tennis ball over the affected area – it may sound strange but it is enormously soothing.
- Ask your husband to massage your lower back and perhaps alternate it with pressure, using a little talc or oil to avoid chafing your skin.
- Rotate your hips in a kind of belly dance.

Gas and air (Entonox)

This is a mixture of half oxygen and half nitrous oxide ('laughing gas'), which you breathe in using a hand-held mask. It makes you feel light-headed and dulls the pain. Because it contains a good quantity of oxygen it is completely harmless to you and your baby, and the gases pass out of your system in between contractions. It takes about 40

Emergency birth

A very fast labour and delivery is known as precipitate labour. Although many mothers-to-be worry that they won't make it to the hospital in time, such births are extremely rare – about one in several hundred. They are more common with a second or subsequent baby, especially if you have already had a very quick labour.

It is important to get medical help as soon as you can. A very rapid labour may be slightly risky for the baby, but she is spared the stress often caused by a long labour and is likely to be born in good condition. The following tips will help if your baby comes in a hurry.

- Stay calm.
- Contact your doctor or midwife, or dial 999 if you can't reach them.
- If there is time, prepare a carrycot for your baby; otherwise a drawer or small box will do until you are able to be more organized.
- Lay plastic, newspaper and old sheets on the floor or bed, and have a clean towel or sheet to wrap the baby in.
- Have other sheets and towels and a sanitary pad handy.
- Cut three lengths of string about 23 cm (9 in.) long with a clean pair of scissors. If you have time, sterilize the string and scissors by boiling for 10 minutes, then wrap them in a clean cloth.
- Kneel with your face down and your bottom in the air, as this may delay the birth for a while.
- If the urge to push becomes irresistible, lie on your back or side and gently support your baby's head as it emerges. Don't pull on either the baby or the cord.
- If the cord is around the baby's neck, gently ease it over her head. Gently remove any membrane that may be covering the baby's face.
- When the baby's body emerges, generally with the next contraction, gently lift her out and lay her over your abdomen. Carefully wipe away any blood or mucus from her mouth and nostrils with a piece of clean sheeting.
- Put the baby to your breast if you wish. This will help stimulate the delivery of the placenta.
- If the baby doesn't breathe at once, hold her with her head lower than her body to drain away any mucus that may be obstructing her passages. *Do not slap her*, but you can splash her with cold water to stimulate an intake of breath.
- You don't have to cut the cord. If it appears before medical help arrives wrap it up and wait for the midwife. If you want to cut the cord, once the baby is breathing, tie it in two places as tightly as you can, about 15 cm and 20 cm (6 in. and 8 in.) away from her navel. Cut it between the two ties, then make another strong tie 10 cm (4 in.) from the navel.
- Wrap your baby in a clean towel or blanket and wait for the midwife to arrive.

seconds for the pain-relieving effect to be felt, so it is best to take several deep whiffs as each contraction starts. You can use it for as long as you like. In practice, most women use it to help them over the end of the first stage of labour. It has the advantage of giving you something to do, so helping to distract you from the pain.

Perhaps the main disadvantage is the face mask, which some women find unpleasantly claustrophobic, and in some hospitals a special mouthpiece is used instead. You will be given instructions on how to use the apparatus during antenatal classes, and a chance to try it out. If you don't have this opportunity, ask your midwife before you have your baby if you can try the equipment so you are familiar with it.

THE BIRTH

SPECIALLY FOR FATHERS

Although the hard, physical work of pushing the baby out falls entirely to the mother, labour is physically and emotionally taxing for you too. You will cope best and be able to help your partner more if you know what to expect. It helps to have been to classes and to have read this book.

The sort of help you give depends on how your wife's labour progresses and on your relationship and personalities. If you have a good idea of what is going on and are aware of the things you can do to help you will be more effective.

Although most fathers are present at the birth these days, you may not want to be there. Perhaps you could be with your wife for some or all of the first stage of labour or, earlier on in her pregnancy, you may be able to help her to find someone else, such as a close friend, relative or antenatal teacher, who would be willing to share her labour.

How can you help?

During the first stage of labour stay with your wife and help her to find the position that is most comfortable and relaxing. During early labour, so long as her waters are still intact, she will probably be happiest at home. She may like to watch television, listen to music or go for a walk. She may find a bath or shower soothing, or she may want you to massage her back, shoulders or abdomen. Remind her to go to the lavatory regularly. If she feels peckish suggest that she has a light snack. Make sure she has plenty of drinks.

As labour progresses your wife will feel the need for quiet concentration. She may like to sink into her own private world. Listening to music on a personal stereo, or listening together, may aid this.

If she has backache she will probably appreciate firm massage, pressure over the painful area, a hot-water bottle or ice pack. Once contractions occur every five minutes or less, make your way to the hospital.

It may help if you breathe with her through contractions. You will also need to interpret her needs to the hospital staff, as by now she won't feel much like talking. If you have already discussed the matter of drugs for pain relief you will be able to help her come to a decision on their use. Be prepared to be flexible. Even if your wife has expressed a desire to do without pain relief she may feel the need for it if labour proves to be difficult or long.

Keep up your encouragement and suggest sips of water. Wipe her brow with a flannel. Reassure her and tell her how well she is doing. Don't get upset if she gets angry and swears at you, as this is a perfectly normal reaction during the transition between first and second stages of labour.

Labour tips for fathers

- Stay calm.
- Help your wife to relax between contractions.
- Encourage her to look into your eyes during contractions to help her concentrate.
- Look to her comfort, anticipate her needs for extra pillows, sips of water, a spoonful of honey.
- Respect your wife's need for silence, and see to it that staff don't interrupt while she is having a contraction.
- Encourage her to let go and groan or sigh if she feels the need.
- Interpret her needs to the medical staff.
- Suggest she tries different positions and moves around if this is possible.
- During the second stage support your wife in any way she wishes.
- Don't become a cheerleader exhorting her to push – let her follow her own natural urge.
- Greet your baby together!

By the way, don't forget to take sandwiches or other snacks to keep up your own strength during labour!

During the second stage encourage your wife to push in accordance with her own instincts. Support her in an upright position or hold her in your arms. If she is keen to give birth in a squatting position you can take her weight by supporting her under the arms from behind. Encourage her to relax between contractions. She may like you to massage her thighs. When the midwife tells her to pant slowly, help her by panting too, so that the baby's head can be eased gently out of the birth canal.

WHAT IF I GO OVERDUE?

Remember your expected date of delivery (EDD) is only an estimate and is not intended to be cast in stone. Some eight out of 10 women deliver within 10 days either side of the EDD, the rest are earlier or later.

More sophisticated methods of testing your baby's well-being enable doctors to be more relaxed about an overdue baby, provided he is healthy.

If you go over your due date, or if at any other time the doctor has reason to suspect your baby is not thriving, you may be asked to keep a kick chart, or to count the number of movements your baby makes and

---

Tips for late arrivals

- Don't pin all your hopes on that magic delivery date – remember it's only an estimate.
- Don't tell the world the day your baby is due – a vague indication of the month will avoid those tiresome 'Are you still around?' comments.
- Arrange for something to do in the days after the EDD – plan a dinner party, an evening with friends, or a short outing (not too far from home!) – to distract yourself.
- Make sure your case is packed and everything is ready for when you go into hospital.
- Don't be too concerned if the medical staff keep changing your EDD. The first ultrasound scan (done at 16–20 weeks) is the most reliable, after which, just like the rest of us, babies grow at different rates.
- Build in some rest and relaxation to your daily routine to prevent you becoming tense and anxious if your EDD comes – and goes.
- Trust your own instincts. If you feel your baby is moving around less than he should, contact your doctor or midwife.
- Remember – all babies are born in the end!

to take the chart along with you the next time you visit the clinic. The doctor will want to check your baby's heart beat to see that it is healthy. A faulty heart beat can be a sign that the baby is running short of oxygen.

A scan will confirm that the baby is well and that the amniotic fluid is sufficient. In some maternity units it is possible to check the blood flow to your baby by means of a Doppler ultrasound scan. If all is well your doctor may decide to let your baby make his appearance in his own good time. Chances are that he's just a born late-starter.

When a baby dies

There are few more devastating experiences than giving birth to a baby who is stillborn or who dies soon after birth. If this happens to you it will take time to come to terms with it.

Stillbirth can be caused by handicap, separation of the placenta, placental insufficiency, some infections that are transmitted across the placenta and complications that arise in labour. In some cases there is no obvious cause.

Studies have shown that many parents who have had this tragic experience find it helpful to be allowed to spend time holding their dead baby and bidding her farewell. A photograph taken at the time can become a treasured reminder of the baby you loved and will help you through the process of grief. It can be especially hard to grieve for a dead baby, as there is not the public recognition that is accorded to the bereaved when an older person dies. It may help if your baby can be given a proper funeral; ask the hospital staff to help you make the necessary arrangements.

After your baby's death you will probably have a strong need repeatedly to relive the experience, in order to try to make some sort of sense of it. Friends and family who love and care for you should try to understand that this is not a morbid preoccupation but part of the work of mourning and letting go.

It usually makes sense to wait until you have been through the grief process before trying for another baby. It may help to talk to others who have undergone the same experience (see page 204 for addresses of associations).

LABOUR AND BIRTH

WHEN LABOUR IS MORE COMPLICATED

INDUCTION

Not so long ago, when induction (artificially starting labour) was a relatively new technique, many doctors would induce simply because a baby was overdue. The reason for this is that the placenta starts to work less efficiently the longer pregnancy continues. At that time it was not possible to measure accurately the functioning of the placenta, so a policy was sometimes put into practice of inducing when a baby was a certain number of days overdue.

Today, thanks to sophisticated techniques for measuring the efficiency of the placenta, you are less likely to be induced simply because your baby is a few days late. What's more, today's methods of induction are much gentler and more natural than they were a few years ago.

When to induce

The main criterion the doctor will use in making a decision is whether the baby is safer inside the womb or not. In practice, this means you will probably be induced in the following situations:

- If you are suffering pre-eclampsia, which reduces blood flow to the placenta and so deprives the baby of sufficient food and oxygen. If the situation is allowed to continue, your health is also at risk.
- If you have high blood pressure, for the same reasons.
- If you are diabetic, in which case your baby could grow extra large and you may have trouble delivering him.
- If your baby is suffering distress.

Is your baby still safe inside the womb?

There are several ways in which the doctor can determine how well your baby is doing. The time-honoured blood pressure and urine checks are, of course, useful. In addition, your baby's heart will be monitored using an external monitor; and you will probably have a scan. You may also be given an oxytocin challenge test, or stress test, to see whether your baby is standing up to his extra time in the womb. This involves stimulating a few contractions, using a hormone drip, and then monitoring the response of your baby's heart. As the uterus contracts your baby's heart beat is affected. Usually it returns to normal at the end of the contraction. If it doesn't, the doctor may decide to induce labour or even to perform a caesarean.

What happens in induction?

If the doctor decides to induce you this can be done in several ways. The routine varies slightly from one hospital to another but one or more of the following methods will usually be used. The same techniques are used to speed up, or accelerate, a labour which is progressing slowly. The most usual first step is to use a special hormone pessary or gel, made of prostaglandins, that softens your cervix in readiness for labour. This is what happens when you go into labour naturally. The pessary or gel is placed high in your vagina against your cervix and is often sufficient on its own to induce labour, if you are ready to give birth. You will usually be admitted to hospital or you may be sent home to await the start of labour. If labour doesn't start within about twelve hours you may be given more pessaries.

Another way of encouraging the uterus to start contracting is by a 'membrane sweep'. This may be done before inserting the hormone pessary. During an internal examination the midwife stretches the cervix slightly and separates the membranes from the neck of the womb.

If these do not spark off labour, your membranes will be broken, using an instrument a bit like a blunt crochet hook. This is called artificial rupture of the membranes, ARM, and causes the baby's head to exert pressure on your cervix, as the water drains away. This will usually cause the onset of contractions. It also enables the doctor to examine the colour of your waters. If they are stained with meconium (your baby's first bowel movement) it is a sign your baby is distressed. Once the membranes are ruptured, the doctor is able to set up an internal monitor.

Finally, if labour has still not started, a hormone drip, containing oxytocin, which is responsible for initiating contractions, will be set up. The hormone is dripped into a vein in your wrist. Contractions begin a few hours after the drip is set up. The length and strength of the contractions are monitored. The drip remains up until after the baby is born.

Can I avoid induction?

Routine induction leads to a higher incidence of caesarean deliveries, and most doctors are reluctant to induce you until you are at least two weeks past your delivery date provided you and the baby are doing well.

If you're ready to go into labour there are one or two tricks you could try to induce yourself. Moving the bowels often has a knock-on effect – hence the old wives' remedy of castor oil and an enema! A hot curry might have the same effect. Regular nipple stimulation sparks off the hormones that cause the uterus to contract, which is why many mothers get 'afterpains' when they breast-feed. Semen contains plenty of the prostaglandins that help soften the cervix. So if an induction has been suggested you might try making love – it can't do any harm, and it may start your labour off.

How will I cope?

Induction may lead to a highly medically managed labour, as it is likely to be shorter and more intense than a natural labour, which progresses through a gradual build-up of painful contractions. You will need plenty of help and support from your husband and those around you. You'll cope better if you understand what is happening and why. Some women manage without any pain relief, but you are more likely to need the aid of drugs if you have an induced labour – and you shouldn't feel ashamed of this.

Coping with a long labour

Normal labour has its own natural pace. A long, slow labour may be easier to cope with than a short, intense one. Experiment with the different positions and postures outlined in these pages, walk about, kneel or squat. Keep up your fluid intake, so you don't get dehydrated. Light snacks, or the occasional spoonful of honey if you don't feel like eating, will help keep up your energy. Relax between contractions.

However, you may need extra help if:

- Despite having contractions, your uterus isn't working properly to open up your cervix. This is called uterine inertia and may be an indication for acceleration or a caesarean.
- There is disproportion between your baby's head and your pelvis, so that the head doesn't engage.
- Your baby is lying in the posterior position and is taking an undue length of time to turn.

EPISIOTOMY

This is a small cut that is made in your perineum (the area of tissue between your vagina and anus), in order to allow more room for the baby's head to emerge and to prevent a ragged tear. It used to be thought that an episiotomy helped prevent prolapse of the pelvic organs (dropped womb) later in life, but several research studies have produced findings that call this conclusion into question. It is now known that a slight tear heals better than an episiotomy and, given time, the birth outlet usually stretches sufficiently to allow the baby through without the need for a cut. Many women who have had an episiotomy complain that it is sore during the weeks after birth, making finding a comfortable position in which to sit and feed difficult. The discomfort can sometimes interfere with love-making even months after birth.

Adopting an upright squatting position and relaxing your pelvic floor muscles may help you to avoid an episiotomy.

Why would I need an episiotomy?
You are likely to need an episiotomy if:

- You have a very quick second-stage labour, so the birth outlet has insufficient time to stretch.

In these cases, you and your baby will be monitored. A check will be kept on your baby's heart rate and a blood sample may be taken from him to see whether he is suffering from lack of oxygen. You may have an X-ray taken to determine whether it is possible for you to give birth normally.

During the second stage of labour delay may be caused by:

- Your uterus not working properly so you are unable to push.
- An epidural.
- A full bladder or rectum.
- A perineum (the area of tissue between your vagina and anus) that is insufficiently soft and relaxed.
- Your baby failing to turn.
- Your baby lying in a difficult position or being abnormally large.
- An abnormality of the baby's head, such as hydrocephalus (water on the brain).

Your doctor will consider all these possibilities and may decide to perform a caesarean or forceps delivery (see pages 146–50).

LABOUR AND BIRTH

- Your baby has a very big head or is lying in an awkward position.
- Your baby is in distress.
- You have to have a forceps delivery (see below).
- Your baby is breech.
- Your baby is premature, in order to avoid undue trauma to his delicate head.
- You are too tired to push the baby out.
- Your tissues are not giving sufficiently, or the midwife thinks you are about to tear badly.

What happens?
The midwife or doctor gives you a local anaesthetic injection to numb the area (this may sting slightly); then makes a small cut, either straight back from the vagina, or in the shape of a J to avoid the anal muscles. After your baby is born, the doctor or midwife sews up the cut. For tips on dealing with post-episiotomy pain see page 175.

Can I avoid an episiotomy?
Some of the following may help you avoid an unnecessary episiotomy:

- Massage your perineum or get your husband to do so, with a mild, non-irritant oil, such as almond, every day during the last three or four weeks of pregnancy. This softens the tissues.
- Practise relaxing your pelvic floor muscles (see page 176).
- During the second stage of labour follow your natural instincts when pushing and adopt a position in which you are comfortable.

FORCEPS OR VENTOUSE DELIVERY

Forceps are shaped like a pair of large, shallow, metal spoons, which lock together around the baby's head and enable the doctor to draw him down and out of the birth canal. Occasionally a vacuum extractor, or ventouse, may be used instead.

Why forceps?
The doctor may decide to use forceps if:

- Your baby is suffering from lack of oxygen after a long second stage.
- You are becoming exhausted by a long, difficult labour.

- You have a medical condition, such as heart or lung disease, or are suffering high blood pressure.
- The baby is breech or lying in a difficult position for birth.
- You have had an epidural or the baby's head has not rotated.
- Your baby is premature.

What happens?

If you have had an epidural there will be no sensation in your perineum. Alternatively, you will be given a local anaesthetic to numb the area. Your feet are placed in stirrups to raise your legs and your bladder is emptied using a catheter. The doctor cleans the birth outlet and gives you an episiotomy. He then gently slides first one forceps blade and then the other around the baby's head and locks them together to protect the baby's skull in the firm 'cage' of the forceps. With the next contraction, you push smoothly as the doctor draws out the baby's head. The forceps are then removed and the rest of your baby's body emerges.

Some doctors prefer to use a vacuum extractor (ventouse), which consists of a small rubber or metal cap attached to a suction tube, to help the baby out, or to help his head rotate into the best position for birth. An episiotomy is first performed. The cup is attached to the baby's head – this may take 10 to 20 minutes. Suction is used to pull the baby downwards, and you can help by pushing with contractions at the same time.

If you've had a forceps delivery your baby may have marks on his face made by the blades for a day or so after the birth. In the case of a ventouse delivery he'll have a bump on the top of his head from the suction, which disappears within a few hours of birth.

CAESAREAN

A caesarean is the process by which the baby is removed from the uterus by means of a surgical cut made through the walls of the abdomen and uterus.

A caesarean section can be a life-saver in certain circumstances. With modern methods of monitoring, which detect when a baby is in distress, and safer anaesthetics, and where a vaginal delivery would cause problems, a caesarean can be a safe alternative.

Why a caesarean?
A caesarean may be carried out if:

- You have dangerously high blood pressure or pre-eclampsia and the placenta is not functioning efficiently.
- The placenta is blocking the entrance to your uterus (placenta praevia), or is shearing away from the wall of the womb (abruptio placenta).
- Your pelvis is too small or misshapen for you to give birth normally.
- Problems occur during labour causing your baby to be distressed (suffer lack of oxygen).
- Your baby is a very low birth weight, and in some cases of handicap.
- You have genital herpes and the sores are open at the time of giving birth.
- Your baby is lying in a position that would make it impossible to give birth normally.
- Despite strong contractions your cervix is failing to open up (inertia).

What happens?
Often a caesarean is planned before you go into labour. This is called an elective caesarean. If you know you are going to have a caesarean, you'll be able to arrange for practical help and back-up when you return home from hospital. If you wish, and depending on the facilities at the hospital, you may be able to have your baby under epidural, in which case you can witness your baby's birth just like any other mother.

If your caesarean is carried out in an emergency, because it becomes vital that your baby is born as quickly as possible during labour, there may be no time for an epidural and you will be given a general anaesthetic instead.

Your pubic hair is shaved from your abdomen, and a catheter is inserted into your bladder to draw off urine. The operation takes five to ten minutes to deliver the baby and another 45 minutes to sew up the uterus and abdomen. A horizontal 'bikini-line' cut is made low on your abdomen, which soon heals, and you can wear a bikini without an unsightly scar. Very occasionally the traditional vertical incision is made. A midwife, and a paediatrician – a doctor who specializes in the care of babies and children – are present to care for your baby as he is born.

An epidural caesarean

1. The midwife cleans your abdomen with antiseptic solution.
2. An epidural is carefully inserted into your back, while you lie curled on your side.
3. The doctor tests that you can't feel any pain.
4. Sterile drapes are placed over your legs and abdomen so you can't see the operation.
5. You'll feel a sensation of pressure as the doctor cuts through the layers of tissue.
6. The doctor gently draws the baby out of the uterus.
7. The midwife sucks any mucus from his nose and mouth.
8. Your first cuddle with your baby.
9. The paediatrician will be present to weigh and measure your baby, and check him over to see that he is healthy.
10. The doctor stitches you up again, or metal clips may be used to seal the wound.

Recovery after a caesarean

If you have had a caesarean your hospital stay will be longer than it would have been after a normal delivery. You will probably stay in for a week to 10 days. After three or four days the dressings will be removed from the wound. The deeper layers of internal stitches will dissolve of their own accord. The stitches on the skin of the abdomen, or clips if used, will be removed towards the end of the first week.

For the first day or so you will feel weak, and probably nauseous from the anaesthetic (if you had a general anaesthetic). Your abdomen will feel bruised and sore. Hold it firmly by placing one hand over the other as you move around to ease discomfort. Try to walk tall, as this will be more comfortable. Wind is sometimes a problem, as an operation tends to slow down the digestive system. Gentle massage may help. The physiotherapist should visit you and offer some suggestions, such as gentle leg circling exercises to keep your circulation on the move. She or he will also help you cough to clear your lungs of fluid that may have accumulated as a result of a general anaesthetic. Try to get out of bed and move around as soon as you can. The staff will help you. This is important to avoid the risk of blood clots. As your uterus shrinks back to its normal size you may experience cramp-like pains. Your antenatal breathing and relaxation may help you deal with these discomforts, and you will be offered pain killers if they are severe. Don't feel you have to suffer in silence. Ask if you think you need an analgesic (pain-relieving drug).

> *Tips to help you cope after a caesarean*
> - Any of the techniques you learnt during pregnancy for easing labour pain may be helpful now. You may also like to ask for pain-relieving drugs, as your scar will be painful.
> - TENS (transcutaneous electrical nerve stimulation), if it is available, may help ease any discomfort you are feeling.
> - You may feel more comfortable with a pillow to support your abdomen as you lie in bed.
> - You'll need help getting into a comfortable position to breast-feed – you may find lying down more comfortable.
> - Rest as much as you can and accept all offers of help.
> - When you bath add a handful of salt to the water to ease the pain of the scar and help it heal.
> - Once you are home avoid climbing stairs until you are feeling stronger. This may take several weeks.
> - You may not feel much like making love for a month or so, which is entirely normal. Find other ways of expressing your love for each other.
> - Contact a caesarean support group for help and advice (see page 204 for addresses).

You've had a major operation, so recovery is bound to take a little longer than after a normal delivery. Recognize this and don't overdo it. You'll need help with heavy jobs and lifting for six weeks after the birth of your baby, and you may be eligible for a home help – enquire about this at your local council offices, or ask your health visitor. It's a good idea to let at least a year elapse before becoming pregnant again, in order to recover your full strength and allow the scar to heal.

Once a Caesar always a Caesar?

If you've had a caesarean you may wonder whether you'll be able to have a normal birth next time. The answer is that you will, unless the problem that caused the need for the first caesarean occurs again. The main reason for another caesarean is that there is insufficient room in your pelvis for your baby's head to descend. Most mothers who have had a caesarean have a normal vaginal delivery the next time around. If you've had a caesarean you'll be advised to have a hospital delivery so that the doctor can keep a careful eye on you during labour.

BREECH BIRTH

If your baby is lying in the breech position labour sometimes starts with some leaking of the waters. This is because the baby doesn't fit so snugly into the pelvis when he is breech. If this happens get in touch with the hospital. There is a danger that the cord could slip down and get trapped between the baby and the cervix, so cutting off his oxygen supply.

If labour begins without any leaking waters, stay upright and move around as much as you can. Once the waters have burst, the best positions to assume to avoid the cord slipping down are kneeling on all fours or lying on your side. Labour will proceed as for a baby who is lying head downwards in the first stage, though it may be slower.

During the second stage, even if the doctor thinks you will be able to have a normal birth, you may be moved to the operating theatre, just in case a caesarean becomes necessary. You may like to squat or go on all fours, or sit in a semi-vertical position supported by your husband or labour companion. Alternatively the doctor may prefer you to lie down with your feet held up in stirrups (this is called the lithotomy position) for ease of access during delivery. The baby should be allowed to pass down the birth canal slowly and gently, without vigorous pushing. Concentrate on breathing calmly, and let your contractions do the work of easing your baby down through your vagina.

Delivery

As your baby's buttocks stretch the birth outlet the doctor will probably do a large episiotomy. He will then deliver the baby's buttocks followed by the legs, though sometimes the baby emerges feet first. The baby then turns and the doctor delivers the head, either by hand or, more often, using forceps. At this point you will probably be told to push. A long, slow push is best.

You may be advised to have an epidural if your baby is breech, in which case you will feel a tugging sensation but no pain as the baby is born.

Will you need a caesarean?

Many obstetricians believe that all breech babies should be delivered by caesarean section for safety. Others argue that in the case of an otherwise uncomplicated breech birth a supported squatting position reduces the chance of cord compression and a consequent cut-off in the oxygen supply. If your pelvis is too small or shaped in such a way that the baby cannot pass through, if your baby is very large or if his legs are extended, a caesarean section will usually be necessary. However, if your baby is of normal size, your pelvic outlet is sufficient, and the baby is lying in a well-flexed position, there is a good chance that you will be able to have a normal delivery.

IF YOUR BABY IS BORN TOO SOON

If your baby is preterm (that is, born before 37 weeks) you are in for an anxious few weeks, or even months. Depending on how early she was born, and her state of health, she will probably need to be nursed in a SCBU (special care baby unit), or – if she is very small and sick – an ICBU (intensive care baby unit).

When birth takes you by surprise in this way it can take extra time to adjust. You may not have had the chance to go to antenatal classes or to sort out any of the practical details to which mothers-to-be usually devote themselves in the last weeks of pregnancy. As a result, you feel bewildered and unprepared. If your baby has to be in hospital while you are at home, you feel cut off from her and may find it hard to believe that you really have a baby.

Most special care baby units make a real effort to involve parents in the everyday care of their tiny babies. You will be encouraged to hold her, change her and give her her feeds, which will help develop the bond between you. Nonetheless, don't be too concerned if it takes you a while to love your baby. Your feelings will gradually grow once you take her home and start getting to know her better.

Preterm babies have three main problems:

- Their lungs are immature, which leads to breathing problems.
- They have little body fat and so find it difficult to maintain a steady temperature.
- If born before 35 weeks they have weak sucking and swallowing reflexes which make feeding from breast or bottle impossible. They have to have small, frequent feeds by means of a tube passed through the nose into the stomach. Sometimes they have to have nutrients dripped straight into a vein.

The SCBU is designed to help your baby overcome these problems. She is nursed in an incubator, which keeps her warm and reduces the amount of sweat evaporation from her skin surface. She may need an

The incubator keeps your baby warm and free from infection, while an intravenous pump supplies her with essential nutrients

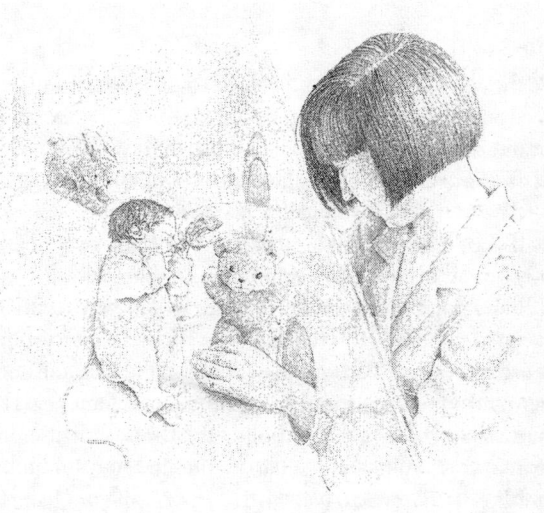

artificial ventilator to enable her to breathe. She will be nursed on an 'apnoea mattress', which sets off an alarm if she develops breathing problems, and she will be fed intravenously or by tube until she is strong enough to suck.

Premature babies are more susceptible to jaundice because their livers are unable to process bilirubin (the yellow pigment produced when red blood cells break down), so they may be nursed under a special light which helps clear the bilirubin from the system. All her other bodily functions, such as heart rate, blood gases and so on, will also be constantly monitored.

Fortunately, premature babies stand an excellent chance of survival. Even those as young as 24 weeks, given expert care and attention, stand a 25–30 per cent chance of pulling through.

If you plan to breast-feed you will need extra patience and perseverance. At first your baby may be tube-fed either with expressed breast milk or a special premature formula. As she becomes stronger you can start to put her to the breast. The midwives will help you. At first your baby will tire easily. Have patience and persevere. You may be able to use the hospital's electric breast pump to build up a milk supply until your baby is strong enough to suck.

As soon as your baby is feeding well, gaining weight and able to maintain her body temperature you will be able to take her home.

Going home

Although you are naturally eager to take your baby home, you may be anxious too. The SCBU may arrange for a special nurse to visit you at home in the first few days and liaise with your local midwife, health visitor and GP. All these experts are there to help you so don't hesitate to contact them if you feel at all worried.

If your baby weighs less than 2.2 kg (5 lb.) you'll probably have to buy or make a few extra small items of baby clothes and cut down some full-size nappies, as the normal size will swamp her. Keep your baby's room at a steady 70°F (21°C). You'll need to feed your premature baby more often than you would a full-term baby. If she doesn't wake and demand a feed you should pick her up and feed her. Don't let her go more than three hours without a feed. She will also probably need extra iron and vitamins, which can be prescribed by your doctor.

It's only natural to feel a little anxious if your baby has had an unsteady start in life. However, the vast majority of premature babies cope well. Your baby may be more prone to coughs and colds during her first year or so. Her prematurity won't affect her mental development, although you can expect her to be a little behind in her developmental milestones for one or two years. Allow her the number of weeks she was born early when calculating what she should be doing. There are various support agencies and services you can turn to for practical help if you have a premature baby (see page 203 for addresses).

Part III

YOU AND YOUR NEW BABY

Your new baby

The first meeting
Your baby may be delivered straight on to your abdomen for you to stroke and caress or he may be handed to you wrapped in a towel to cuddle and admire. In whatever way you greet him there is something magical about those first few moments. You feel a mixture of awe, wonder and amazement that this tiny creature belongs to you. You may laugh or weep, or you may feel a sense of unreality, as if this isn't really happening to you. Accept all these conflicting emotions and don't be afraid to give rein to your laughter or tears.

At some point after the birth the midwife will want to check your baby over. Once this examination has been carried out and you are cleaned up, you and your husband will probably be allowed to spend some time together with your new baby. You will probably want to undress your baby and marvel at his perfection. If you are breast-feeding you may like to let him suckle for a while at your breast, either on the delivery table or afterwards. You'll probably feel, despite his somewhat squashed appearance, that he is the most beautiful baby in the world. Don't worry if you feel none of these things. You may need a while to recover, especially if you've had a long, difficult labour. Some mothers fall instantly and irrevocably in love with their babies. Others find it takes a while for love to grow. You'll find your feelings of attachment blossom as you spend more time with your baby and get to know him.

Life in the outside world
Just as you have to get used to being a mother, so your new baby has to adjust from the warm, wet comfort of the world he has known inside you, to the cold, noisy outside environment.

The biggest change is the switch in his circulatory system. While he was inside the womb his blood flowed in and out via his lifeline, the placenta, which acted as his 'lungs' taking in oxygen and passing out carbon dioxide into your blood stream. Your baby's first breath stimulates changes in his circulation: the blood vessels in the umbilicus close down and his own system takes over. He is an independent human being. But he still needs all the love and care you can give him to ease his existence in the outside world.

For the first time he has to breathe through his nose. He's already practised breathing movements while in the womb but he's still a beginner. You'll notice that his breathing seems irregular. Even more alarmingly, sometimes he appears to stop breathing altogether for a second or so.

He has to become used to the changeable temperature of the world outside. As his heat-regulating mechanism still isn't fully operational, it's up to you to see that he stays warm.

In the womb your baby's food came 'pre-digested'. He obtained his nutrients from your blood via the placenta. Now he has to suck, swallow, digest, absorb and excrete food all by himself. Fortunately, he is endowed with certain reflexes (see pages 161–2) that enable him to stay well nourished. The special, highly nourishing and easily digested form of milk – colostrum – produced by your breasts help to ease him over his first few days of life.

Your baby will pass his first bowel movement within 24 hours of birth. It is greenish-black and sticky. This meconium, as it is called, is the residue of mucus and other products he swallowed in the womb. Over the next few days his motions will become soft and yellow. A bottle-fed baby's stools are slightly more formed than those of a breast-fed baby.

A world of sensations

From the start your baby's senses are highly developed. He'll recognize your voice and that of his father even as you lie on the delivery bed. If he is crying and he hears your voices he may even calm down and turn his head as if trying to locate the familiar sounds. Within a few days he will recognize your unique smell. And though his eyesight is not as acute as an adult's, and he has trouble in focusing, he will recognize your face when he is just two days old. Your baby will love you to pick him up and talk to him. He relies on you to introduce him to the strange new world in which he finds himself.

Your baby's appearance

At birth your midwife or doctor will examine your baby to make sure all is well. She will probably clear his nose and mouth of any mucus and free the air passages so that he can breathe. She will clamp and cut the umbilical cord, then weigh and measure him. If you are in hospital, he will be given a name tag, detailing his name, sex, birth date and weight, which will be wrapped around his wrist.

Apgar score The Apgar score is a method used to measure your baby's well-being, and how well he has stood up to the stress and strain of birth. One minute after birth the midwife will assess by simple observation five vital signs to see that your baby is fit and well. These are: heart rate, breathing, skin colour, muscle tone, and response to stimulation. Each vital sign is assigned 2, 1 or 0 points, and these are added up. If the baby scores between 8 and 10 points it shows he is in good condition at birth. A very low score indicates the need for resuscitation. The Apgar score is checked again five minutes later, and at five-minute intervals after that in the case of a baby who needs help in starting to breathe.

Most healthy babies have a bluish tinge to their hands and feet for several hours after birth, as a result of their sluggish circulation. It's of no importance.

Although you are delighted with your new baby, you may find his appearance a little strange. His head seems large and wobbly. His tummy is round and barrel-shaped. His arms and legs seem scrawny and delicate. Over the next few weeks, however, he'll begin to acquire the chubby, rosy look usually associated with babies.

He may have patches of greasy white vernix in the creases of his skin, or his skin may be dry and peeling. There may be traces of fine down (lanugo) on his shoulders and back. He may have a mop of hair or be quite bald. His eyes are slate grey. Later they will change to their permanent colour.

Head Your baby's head may seem oddly shaped from the moulding of the bones that allowed him to pass down the birth canal. Sometimes he will have a strange lump on the top of his head. These lumps and bumps will gradually disappear over the next few days. Your baby has two 'soft spots', called fontanelles, at the front and back of his head where the bones of his skull have not yet joined. These allow his skull to grow. Gradually over the next 18 months the fontanelles, which are covered by a strong membrane, will grow smaller and eventually close.

Face You may notice small red 'stork bites', or birthmarks called capillary naevi, on his eyelids and the bridge of his nose or the back of his neck, which will gradually fade over the next few months. He may also have tiny pearly spots, called milia or 'milk spots', over the bridge of his nose. They are caused by blocked skin glands and will disappear as his system starts to work more effectively. Most skin blemishes gradually fade. Permanent birthmarks which are flat or raised may be present at birth or may appear during the first few months afterwards.

Your baby's eyes may wander and he may appear to squint. This is simply because he can't yet focus both eyes at once. You'll also notice that your baby doesn't cry tears until he is about a month old.

Genitals If your baby is a boy his testicles will be in the scrotum. You won't be able to push his foreskin back, as it is still fused to the tip of the penis. It will gradually separate during the first few years of his life. Both boys and girls may have swollen genitals at first. A girl baby may have a slight blood loss, like a period, as a result of your hormones being withdrawn at birth. She may also have a thick white vaginal discharge. Both are normal and nothing to worry about.

Breasts Some babies have enlarged breasts and may even produce a little milk (witches' milk), as a result of the withdrawal of your hormones. There is no need to do anything about this, and your baby's breasts will gradually become flatter over the next few weeks.

Skin Newborn babies' skin often flares up in rashes and spots that seem most alarming but usually last only a short time. Nettle rash (neonatal urticaria) is a blotchy red rash with a raised yellow centre. It often occurs in the first week and disappears within a day or so. The traditional red heat rash is also common and passes off as your baby cools down. A bottle-fed baby may be susceptible to nappy rash. Thorough cleansing when you change his nappy and exposing his bottom to air will help clear it up, or the hospital staff may be able to suggest a cream you could use.

NEW BABY CHECK-UPS

During your hospital stay your baby will be given a thorough examination by a paediatrician, at which you will usually be able to be present. If you give birth at home the baby will be checked over by your GP. So what will the doctor do, and why?

As the baby is undressed, the doctor will observe the way she moves and how alert she seems. He or she will examine all the baby's external organs – her skin, limbs, eyes – to check that they are normal, and will listen to her heart to see that it is beating strongly. Often the doctor will pick up a slight heart murmur, but this is usually quite harmless and does not mean your baby is in any way abnormal. Your baby's breathing will be checked, too.

The doctor will also test for congenital dislocation of the hip (CDH), which, if detected, is completely curable at this early stage. If the test proves positive – and a girl is more likely to be affected than a boy – the baby will have to wear a special splint for about six to 12 weeks.

The doctor will weigh and measure your baby and ask you how she is feeding. Your baby may lose up to 10 per cent of her birth weight in the first three days after birth, but she will normally have regained her birth weight by the 10th day. After that, for the first three months she will gain approximately 200 g (7 oz.) a week.

REFLEXES

All babies are born with a set of reflexes. The doctor will check some of these to ensure the baby's nervous system is working properly. Gradually, over the next few months, these reflexes fade, to be replaced by deliberate voluntary movements.

The sucking reflex
Your baby will automatically suck on any object placed in her mouth – she practised sucking her thumb while she was still in the womb.

Rooting reflex
A touch on the side of your baby's cheek or the corner of her mouth will cause her to turn and look for food. This reflex combined with the sucking reflex ensures your baby knows how to feed during the first few days of life.

Grasp reflex
Your baby's fingers – and toes – will automatically grip any object placed in them. Newborn babies can even support their own body weight in this way.

'Moro' or the startle reflex
This is the reaction you will notice if your baby hears a loud noise or is

surprised in any way. She flings open her arms and legs, then slowly clasps them together across her body as though to protect herself.

Walking reflex

If you hold your baby upright with the soles of her feet on a hard surface she will 'step out', as though walking. She will also 'step up' on to a table in the same way if you place her shin against the edge of it.

SCREENING TESTS

During your hospital stay your baby will be screened for certain abnormalities.

Guthrie test

Sometimes known as the 'heel prick test', this involves taking a small blood sample from your baby's heel, to test it for phenylketonuria, a rare condition in which the body is unable to cope with the enzyme phenylalanine, found in food. Left untreated it can cause mental handicap. If detected at this stage your baby can be put on a special diet and will grow normally. The same test is used to check for hypothyroidism (underactivity of the thyroid gland) and diabetes, both of which can be treated.

Meconium test

This may be carried out on your baby's first bowel motion after birth to check for cystic fibrosis, a rare genetic condition caused by an enzyme deficiency. Untreated it can cause permanent damage to the lungs. If detected your baby will be put on a special diet, with vitamin supplements and enzyme replacements.

Establishing feeding

Most mothers have decided how they are going to feed their baby by the time the baby is born. The choices are outlined in the section on feeding (pages 50–53). Much of your stay in hospital, or the first few days after birth if you are at home, will be spent getting feeding established. Don't be afraid to ask the hospital staff or your community midwife to help you at any time, even though they may seem busy.

Solving any problems while there are people there to help you will ease the transition to home life, particularly if you are breast-feeding.

During the first weeks of your baby's life much of your time will be spent feeding him. Newborn babies need feeding little and often. Your baby will be happier and will settle more quickly if you let him decide when he wants to be fed. At first this is likely to be every couple of hours or so. Later on, the interval between feeds extends, until by about his sixth week he is having just six or seven feeds a day.

BREAST-FEEDING

If you've decided to breast-feed you can be sure that you are giving your baby a good start in life. If you are still undecided after you have had your baby, why not give breast-feeding a try? You can always go over to the bottle if you find it doesn't suit you. Don't worry if your baby doesn't take to the breast straight away. Let him lick and nuzzle your nipple, and try again later. Your baby only needs a small amount of colostrum in order to survive. This is because it is a highly concentrated food, specially designed for the first few days after birth. Healthy babies who are fed on demand usually want just three to five feeds in the first couple of days, followed by an increase in demand on the third or fourth day after birth, when milk starts to be produced. The number of feeds will fall over the next week or so.

There's no need for your baby to be given anything other than colostrum in these first few days. Although if you are ill, or exhausted after labour, your baby may be given a small feed of water and glucose to tide him over while you catch up on your rest.

Even if your baby has been given bottle-feeds for a few days, for example if either of you is too ill for breast-feeding, you will still be able to breast-feed. If you have to be separated from your baby you can learn how to draw off (express) your milk to be fed to your baby in a bottle or tube (if your baby is premature).

When to start

You can put your baby to your breast while still on the delivery bed. Your baby is born with a strong instinct to suck. Unless he is ill or drowsy from the effects of drugs he will probably latch on vigorously. His sucking will stimulate contractions and help your body deliver the placenta.

Your baby's sucking reflex is at its strongest about 30 minutes after birth. At first he will probably just nibble and lick your nipple, but after a little while he will start sucking.

This first feed will help promote the bond between you and your baby. Your baby will also get the benefit of the colostrum that is produced by your breasts during pregnancy and in the first few days. This fluid is not only full of nutrients, but it provides your baby with some of your antibodies, so helping him to resist infection. Colostrum also helps your baby's gut in making it resistant to harmful bacteria.

Putting your baby to the breast

To begin with, your baby seems impossible to handle, and you are bound to feel clumsy and awkward. Your midwife will help you put your baby to the breast correctly and you'll soon learn how to do it. Sit comfortably on the bed or on a chair. You might find it helpful to have a stool beneath your feet to bring your lap up to the right height; or a pillow across your lap or beneath your elbow to support your baby.

Let your baby nuzzle and lick your nipple. If you stroke the side of his mouth with your nipple, he will turn his head and open his mouth wide. As he does so, slip the nipple and most of the surrounding brown area (the areola) into his mouth. This will prevent sore nipples and ensure he is in the best position to get the milk effectively. A baby gets milk not just by sucking but by squeezing with his gums on the milk sacs lying beneath the areola.

How long should I let him feed?

There's no need to time your baby on the breast. He will stop sucking when he has had enough. At first he may want to spend only a few minutes sucking. Later the length of feeds will increase. So long as you don't become sore there is no need to limit his sucking time. Your baby will suck in bursts: fast at the beginning of the feed, and with long, slow sucks later on. When he has finished one side he will usually stop sucking and let go of the nipple. Breast-fed babies love sucking, and many spend a long time sucking just for the enjoyment of it. Putting the baby to the breast for comfort is an almost guaranteed cure if he is crying. Nevertheless, once you are home it probably won't be convenient to let him suck for a long time at every feed. Your baby gets most of the milk in the first five minutes on each breast. At first he gets the thirst-quenching 'foremilk'. Towards the end of the feed he gets the more satisfying 'hindmilk', which helps him to last longer between feeds.

Taking your baby off the breast

If your baby doesn't stop sucking on his own, you can remove the baby from the breast by slipping a (clean) little finger into the corner of his mouth to break the suction. Alternatively, pull his chin down or depress your breast slightly. Whatever you do, don't just pull or you will make yourself sore.

How often should I feed?

There's no need to clock-watch when you breast-feed. Babies thrive best if they are fed whenever they seem hungry (on demand). In the early weeks this may be every two to three hours because breast milk is so perfectly suited to your baby's digestion.

Breast-feeding works by supply and demand. Whenever your baby sucks, hormones are released that stimulate your breasts to produce more milk. So the more often you feed, the more milk your breasts produce. Your baby doesn't need complementary feeds (extra feeds of formula from a bottle) as this will interfere with the establishment of supply and demand. By the time your baby is six weeks old your milk supply will be producing the exact amount your baby needs. If you need to step up the supply at any time, because your baby doesn't seem satisfied, you can do so simply by increasing the number of feeds. After a day or so your supply will have caught up with his increased demand and you can go back to the number of feeds you were giving.

Let-down reflex

When your baby sucks at the breast hormones are released, causing the milk to rush from the back of your breasts, where it is made and stored, and squirt out through your nipples. This is called the let-down reflex. You probably won't feel it straight away if you are a first-time mother, but you will eventually recognize it as a warm, prickling sensation that fades after a few moments. You may notice that milk drips from the other breast as your baby is feeding. You may also notice that you can bring on the let-down reflex simply by thinking about your baby or hearing your baby cry.

Getting started

Breast-feeding is natural but, like any other new skill, it takes time and practice to learn it. If you encounter difficulties in the early days don't worry – given patience, perseverance and plenty of encouragement, you'll soon overcome them.

Engorgement On the third or fourth day after birth, when your milk comes in, your breasts may become hot, heavy and swollen. This condition, called engorgement, is caused not only by the milk but by an increased blood flow to the area. With care it should pass off within a day or so.

You can help by feeding your baby little and often to keep the milk ducts clear. Expressing a little milk (your midwife will show you how) may help to keep the milk flowing and make it easier for your baby to grasp the nipple. Wear a good supporting bra, and apply ice packs or cold flannels to your breasts to reduce swelling and make you feel more comfortable.

Sore nipples Many mothers, especially those with fair hair or skin, experience some slight soreness in the early days after birth. Positioning your baby correctly on the nipple will help to prevent soreness. If you do become sore, dry your nipples carefully after each feed and expose them to the air as much as you can. It may help to apply a jet of warm air to them from a hair dryer or blow heater or, if it is summer, to do a spot of topless sunbathing.

Wash your nipples in water only, as soap can be an irritant. You don't need to wash them at every feed. Apply a cream or spray to alleviate the soreness – your midwife will be able to recommend one.

While your nipples are sore keep feeds as short as possible. Start feeding on the least sore side first and vary the feeding position so that your baby doesn't exert pressure on the same point of the nipple each time. Some mothers find that the soreness is eased by a drop of milk left to dry on the nipple after a feed.

If the nipple cracks you may need to rest it for a day and express the milk to be fed to your baby by bottle or spoon. When you feed again, start each feed on the less sore side.

Avoid putting your baby to the breast purely for comfort and limit his sucking time to 10 minutes on each side until your nipples have recovered. If your baby needs to suck a lot, try giving him a dummy.

Giving a breast-feed

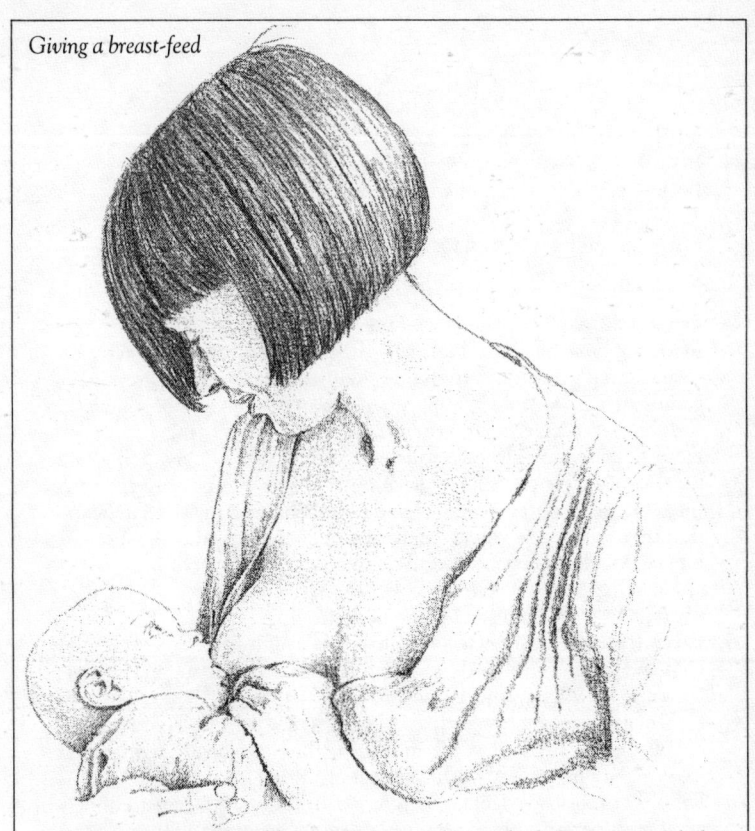

1. Settle into a comfortable position, on a chair or bed. Support your baby's neck in the crook of your arm.
2. Lean slightly forward and 'tease' your baby's lips open with your nipple.
3. When he opens his mouth wide slide the nipple and most of the darker surrounding area into his mouth.
4. Watch the little muscles just above his ears to check they are moving. This will show that he is sucking correctly. Listen to him sucking and swallowing.
5. Let your baby pause from time to time. Each feed has its natural rhythm and breast milk flows in waves, not continuously like milk from a bottle.
6. When either of you has had enough, slip your little finger into the corner of his mouth to remove him from the nipple.

Winding. Not all babies need winding after a feed. If the wind hasn't come up in a few seconds, you can lay him down. He'll probably pass the wind in his sleep.

True or false?

1. If I have small breasts I won't be able to breast-feed my baby.
2. Whenever my baby cries he must be hungry.
3. If I feed my baby on demand he'll get spoilt.
4. Breast-feeding will make me tired.
5. Both breasts must be emptied at each feed.
6. You can't breast-feed when your baby has teeth.
7. My breast milk is too thin for my baby.

In fact, all these are examples of breast-feeding myths.

1. **False** The shape and size of your breasts has nothing to do with your success at breast-feeding. Normally the breasts are made up of fatty tissue, and it's this that determines their size. During pregnancy milk glands are laid down. The supply depends on the amount of stimulation your breasts receive, not on their size.
2. **False** Babies don't always cry just because they are hungry. Some babies, for example, always cry for a few minutes before they go to sleep. Inexperienced mothers often regard their babies' crying as an indication that they aren't receiving enough milk. Very rarely is this the case. So long as your baby appears healthy, has a wet nappy every time you change him, and soft yellow stools, and is gaining about 114–170 g (4–6 oz.) a week, you can be sure he is thriving.
3. **False** If you feed your baby on demand, he will learn to trust you. Demand feeding ensures that you build up a good milk supply for your baby and he will become less erratic in his habits.
4. **False** Breast-feeding isn't tiring. Having a new baby is. Try to get a couple of early nights a week, and during the time you are giving night feeds make sure you rest with your feet up during the day.
5. **False** Let your baby decide when he's had enough. At some feeds he will want more than at others – just as sometimes you want a snack, sometimes a three-course meal.
6. **False** Your baby doesn't use his teeth to feed. You can continue to breast-feed for as long as you are both happy with it.
7. **False** Breast milk looks thinner and more watery than cow's milk, but it is the right quality for your baby. The precise make-up of breast milk varies from mother to mother but, unless you are severely malnourished, it is always nutritionally adequate.

EXPRESSING YOUR MILK

Expressing means drawing off the milk in your breasts by hand or with a breast pump. Learning the simple techniques of expression can help make breast-feeding more flexible. You can express a bottle of milk and leave it to be fed to your baby by whoever is looking after him when you go out, knowing that he is still getting the benefit of your milk in your absence.

Expressing is also useful if your baby is unable to feed from the breast because he is premature or too ill to suck. These babies benefit especially from breast milk, and it can help you feel you are doing something for your baby at a time when you may feel especially helpless. If your baby is premature you will need to express at least four or five times a day to ensure a good supply.

To express by hand

Before starting to express, relax. This will help your milk flow more readily.

1. Have a wide bowl or sterile container ready.
2. Wash your hands. Firmly but gently stroke your breast several times from the outside towards the nipple. This helps move milk down the ducts into the reservoirs which lie below the areola.
3. Place your thumb and forefinger on either side of the areola, with your thumb at the top and your fingers underneath. Using a firm, rhythmic pressure squeeze gently until drops of milk appear at the nipple. After a while you will feel the tingle of the let-down reflex and milk will start to spurt out easily.
4. Continue squeezing gently but firmly for about five minutes. Then move your fingers round so that they rest on either side of the areola, to ensure that all the milk sacs are emptied. Continue for another five minutes.
5. Repeat on the other side. Then go back to the first breast and carry out the procedure again to ensure that as much milk is expressed as possible.

It may take a while to learn to express by hand, but once you do so you will find it useful.

To express by pump

There are several varieties of breast pump on the market. You may be able to borrow one from one of the breast-feeding organizations for temporary use (for example if you have to take the baby off the breast for any reason). The old-style bulb pump may be harsh on your nipples if they are cracked, and it can also harbour germs because of the way it is designed. A useful type of hand pump is the syringe action type, which has a curved plastic cup designed for different sizes of breast. Electric pumps are available in most maternity units, and are the most useful way of collecting milk if you have to express frequently, for example if your baby is very premature.

1. Put the pump together according to the instructions.
2. Place the cup over the nipple to form an airtight seal.
3. Gently draw the cylinder away and downwards. You will see the nipple being drawn backwards and forwards and after a few minutes milk will start to flow.
4. Remove the pump, and fit a teat so the milk can be fed to your baby.

Storing expressed milk

- Put the milk straight into the refrigerator. It can be safely stored for 48–72 hours.
- You can store breast milk in the freezer for six months. Use a sterile plastic container – not glass, which could break.

Building up your milk supply

The following measures will usually boost your milk supply in a day or so. If your baby still doesn't seem satisfied or is losing weight see your health visitor.

- Feed more frequently for a day or so.
- Make sure your baby is properly positioned on the breast.
- Have plenty of rest and relaxation.
- Eat well.
- Gradually cut out any bottle-feeds that you are giving in addition to the breast (complementary feeds).
- Have plenty to drink.
- Eat foods high in B vitamins, for example wholemeal bread, liver and yeast extract, or try Brewer's yeast, which is available at health food shops.

BOTTLE-FEEDING

Make feed times special times when you cuddle your baby close and talk to him. Although one of the advantages of bottle-feeding is that other people can give feeds, try not to make a habit of handing your baby around from one person to another. It will make him feel insecure. Of course, your baby's father will enjoy giving feeds, and you can encourage him to share in feeding right from the start.

Feeding your baby

Make feed times happy occasions and never leave your baby propped on his own with his bottle. Not only will he be lonely, he could also choke.

1. Warm the bottle by holding it under the tap, standing it in hot water or using a bottle warmer.
2. Shake a few drops on the inside of your wrist to check the temperature. It should feel comfortably warm.
3. Find a comfortable place to sit and settle with your baby held in the crook of your arm.
4. Slightly loosen the cap of the bottle to stop the teat collapsing as your baby sucks.
5. Tilt the bottle until the teat is full of milk.
6. Make sure the teat is well back in your baby's mouth.
7. Let your baby set the pace. He may want to stop and look around.
8. Sit him upright or support him against your shoulder to get his wind up. If none comes up within a few minutes he probably doesn't need to burp.

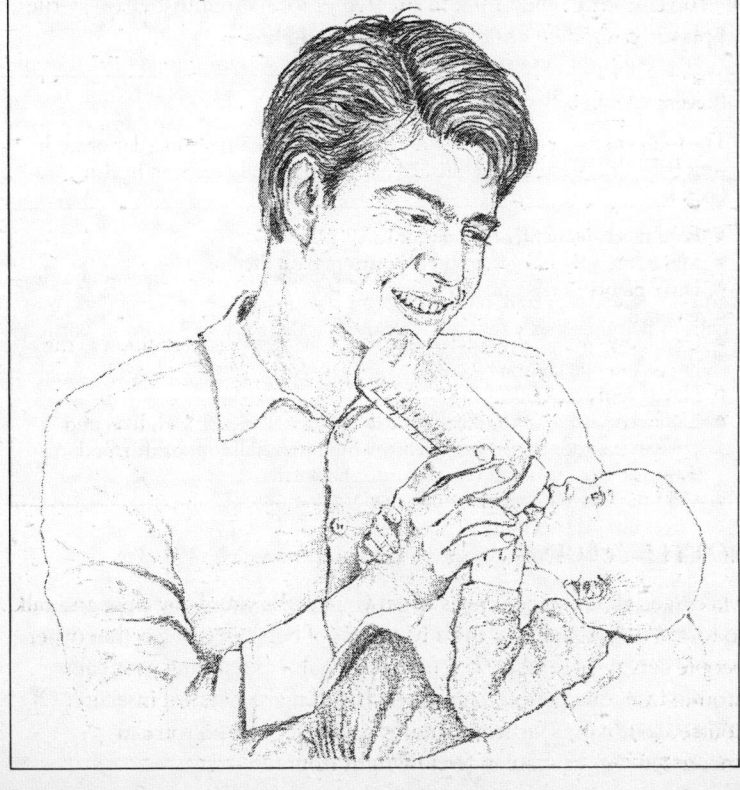

Which milk?

There are many types of milk powder available, and your midwife or health visitor will gladly advise you of a suitable one. A newborn baby needs a highly modified or humanized formula, which, like breast milk, is quickly digested. This consists of skimmed cow's milk, whey, fatty acids and lactose (a type of milk sugar), together with essential vitamins and minerals. You can feed your baby with this on demand, just as if you were breast-feeding. Your baby will thrive on this formula alone for the first three or four months. In fact, milk is the most suitable food for your baby for six months to a year, although your baby will, of course, need some solids in addition to milk feeds by six months.

How many feeds?

Your baby will thrive best if you feed him on demand. At first he will want about seven small feeds a day. Later on he will gradually reduce the number of feeds. A rough guide to the amount your baby needs is 150 ml (5 fl. oz.) per kilogram (2 lb.) of body weight per day. Work out the total amount and divide it by the number of bottles he has. This is not a rigid rule, of course: occasionally your baby will want more, or he may not want to finish his bottle.

Making up a bottle-feed

You will find it is most convenient to make up a whole day's supply of bottles and store them, covered in the fridge, until you need them. Never give your baby milk from a bottle that has been used. If there is milk left in the bottle after the feed, pour it away.

1. Wash your hands
2. Boil a kettle and allow it to cool a little.
3. Take the bottle out of the sterilizing unit and shake off excess solution.
4. Pour the exact amount of water into the bottle.
5. Add the exact amount of milk powder. Do not pack down the powder. Level it off with a knife in the scoop provided.
6. Put on the lid and shake the bottle until the powder is mixed in completely.
7. When you are ready to feed the baby, take the teat out of the sterilizing unit and put it on the bottle.

Sterilizing

Scrupulous hygiene is essential when you are bottle-feeding. Any traces of milk left on bottles or teats are a breeding ground for germs and can give your baby diarrhoea and vomiting.

1. Wash out the bottles thoroughly in warm, soapy water. Use a bottle brush to ensure that no traces of milk are left inside.
2. Clean the teats by rubbing them with salt to get rid of milk and mucus. Rinse thoroughly under running water to clean off the salt.
3. Rinse bottles and teats in clear, clean water.
4. Fill sterilizing unit with water.
5. Add tablets or sterilizing solution. If using tablets make sure they are completely dissolved.
6. Immerse bottles and teats and any other equipment (not metal) in the solution, making sure there are no air bubbles.
7. Cover the unit and leave for at least three hours.
8. Never take the bottles out before they have soaked for the required length of time.

Testing the teat

The milk should drip in steady, fast drops when you hold the bottle upside down. If the hole is too small, heat a needle and place it in the hole in the teat to widen it.

YOUR BODY

In the six weeks after birth all the changes that took place in your system during pregnancy are slowly reversed. Your uterus, ovaries, cervix, blood pressure and bowel and bladder functions gradually go back to normal.

Try not to be impatient if it takes a while to recover your old shape – after all, it took nine months to grow your baby.

Your breasts

As soon as you have given birth hormones are released that cause your breasts first to produce colostrum and then, after three or four days, breast milk. If you are breast-feeding, your baby's sucking will continue to stimulate milk production until she is completely weaned. If you are bottle-feeding, your breasts will stop producing milk and gradually return to normal.

Your breasts may never return to the shape and size they were before you had a baby – irrespective of how you decide to feed. During pregnancy the fatty padding in your breasts is replaced by milk-making glands. After you stop feeding, or earlier if you choose to bottle-feed, this process gradually goes into reverse. Even so, you will probably find your breasts are less firm than they were before. You may have developed stretch marks on them, although these will slowly fade to almost invisible silvery streaks.

Tips to help firm your breasts

- Splash your breasts with cold water after having a bath.
- Circle your arms forwards and backwards vigorously every day to exercise the pectoral muscles.
- Clasp your hands together and, with your arms raised to chest height, press rhythmically and release. You should see the muscles that support your breasts twitch as you do this.
- Lie flat on your back and, holding a pair of light weights (2 kg or 4 lb.), or perhaps a couple of tins if you don't have weights, raise your arms in front of you until your hands meet, then slowly lower them again.
- Wear a good supporting bra for as long as you breast-feed.

Your abdomen

Although your stomach will seem miraculously flatter once you have given birth, you will be left with slack muscles and stretched skin. Practising gentle postnatal exercises – you'll be given a sheet of them by the midwife or physiotherapist – will help.

Your uterus

Gradually over the six weeks following the birth your uterus will shrink to its former shape and size. It should be below your pelvic brim by the 10th day (its position when you were about three months pregnant). The midwife will check every day until the 10th day to ensure that it is contracting as it should. For three or four days after the birth, mothers of second and subsequent babies may feel quite strong afterpains or contractions as the uterus shrinks, especially during breast-feeding when hormones are released that stimulate the uterus to contract. To ease discomfort practise your antenatal relaxation exercises, or if these are not sufficient ask for a pain killer.

Vaginal losses or lochia

You will have a blood loss like a heavy period after you have had your baby. For the first three or four days it is bright red, changing slowly to a pink then yellowish-brown by the end of the first week or so. If the lochia suddenly turns red again after the first week tell the doctor as it could be a sign that you have retained bits of placenta and these could cause a haemorrhage. You will be given a course of tablets to encourage the uterus to squeeze out any leftover material. If the treatment doesn't work you may have to go back to hospital for a dilatation and curettage (D & C) to clean out your uterus.

Stitches

If you've had a tear or a cut you will feel sore for a few days. Walking, sitting, coughing, passing a bowel motion or anything else that puts pressure on the stitches may hurt. Sitting on a rubber ring may help to take the pressure off the stitches, and practising your relaxation exercises will ease the discomfort. Once basic healing has taken place smooth in a mild ointment or cream (a good one is calendula, available from health food stores, or ask your midwife to suggest one). A handful of salt in the bath water will help heal the bruised tissues, and a warm jet of air from a hair dryer is soothing and will speed recovery. A fine spray of warm or cold water from a bidet or shower head is also soothing and healing. An ice pack (wrap ice cubes in a clean flannel) placed against your perineum will bring relief, or soak your sanitary pad in witch hazel.

Using the lavatory

Your bladder may have taken quite a battering during birth as your baby's head pressed on it, and it may be slightly sluggish. Even so, you should pass water within eight hours of giving birth. If you fail to do so you will need to have a catheter inserted to draw off the urine. Urine left in your bladder could render you more liable to develop a urine infection (cystitis), so make sure you have plenty to drink. If you are breast-feeding you will probably feel desperately thirsty when you feed anyway. Drink lemon barley water, as this will make your urine less likely to sting. If you have difficulty passing water try doing it in a warm bath or sitting on a bidet. Contract and relax your pelvic floor muscles, as you learnt in antenatal classes. And try the good old wives' remedy of running the tap when you go to the lavatory.

Your bowels, too, may seem a bit reluctant to function again after birth. If you have had stitches you may be afraid of the discomfort or that the stitches will burst – they won't. Take a mild pain killer, such as paracetamol, relax as you sit on the lavatory, hold a clean pad over your stitches and apply gentle pressure as you bear down. Squatting rather than sitting on the lavatory may help, or squat over a bed pan or potty.

If constipation is a problem have plenty to drink (a teaspoon of lemon juice in a full tumbler of warm water taken first thing in the

---

Don't neglect your pelvic floor

One set of muscles that is important for your health and well-being is the pelvic floor muscles. These are the invisible muscles which support the organs of your pelvic cavity – the bladder, uterus and back passage. The muscles will have become stretched as a result of childbirth and you need to exercise them just as you would other parts of your body to get them back into shape. Strong muscles in this area reduce the chance of prolapse (dropped womb) later in life and of leaking drops of urine under pressure (stress incontinence). They can also improve your sex life. Because these muscles are invisible it is easy to forget to exercise them, but you should aim to keep them well-toned in order to avoid the problems mentioned above.

The muscles of the pelvic floor form a figure of eight, which supports your anus, vagina and urethra. It's easy to practise tightening and releasing these muscles by imagining that you are in urgent need of passing water. Try to build regular flexing of these muscles into your day. You should aim to do about 100 every day. Don't worry if at first you find you can't hold the muscles tightened for long. At first it will be quite difficult but the muscles will gradually become stronger as you practise. You can also practise stopping and starting the urine flow when you visit the lavatory.

A useful way to practise pelvic floor tightening is to imagine that the area is a lift. Gradually draw it up to the first floor, and then hold for a few seconds. Then move to the second floor, and so on, until the muscles are tight. Gradually release them down until they reach the bottom floor. End the exercise by drawing in the muscles again to the first floor. As the muscles grow stronger you will be able to hold them for longer periods. Rest between these exercises to avoid the muscles getting over-tired.

Another good, and pleasurable, way of exercising is to squeeze your partner's penis by tightening your internal muscles when you make love.

As well as these specific exercises, any other regular exercise helps to tone the pelvic muscles and keep them in trim.

morning is said to be helpful), and eat a high-fibre diet. Hospital menus often leave a lot to be desired so get your husband to bring in fresh and dried fruit and some bran cereal.

It is best to avoid taking laxatives, especially if you are breast-feeding as they can upset your baby's tummy. Your midwife may suggest you use suppositories or a natural laxative.

If piles are troublesome your doctor can prescribe a cream or a stool-coating pessary to ease discomfort.

Mood swings

You may find your emotions swing violently from elation to depression in the early days. You probably feel more exhausted than you ever remember feeling in your life; you may find you sleep only fitfully and that you have especially vivid dreams or nightmares. On the third or fourth day after the birth you may feel particularly tearful – this is the famous fourth-day blues. These mood changes are all perfectly usual. They're partly a result of the enormous hormonal upheaval that follows birth; and partly to do with all the other changes that are going on in your life right now. Overnight you have become a mother. If you are in hospital you are having to adapt to a strange environment with

---

How long will it take me to get my figure back?

Immediately after birth your figure may seem rather flabby. This is entirely to be expected and it will take six to nine months before your figure returns completely to normal.

Breast-feeding will help you to regain your former shape and firmness by using up the pads of fat laid down during pregnancy as stores for your baby. However, you may not lose all the extra weight until after you have stopped breast-feeding. It is best not to diet until you have finished breast-feeding, as it could affect the milk supply. Eat sensibly and cut out cakes, and sweet or fatty foods. If you are still overweight you can go on a calorie-counted diet after you have weaned your baby.

Of course, dieting is not the only way to regain your figure. You also need to firm up your stretched muscles with exercise. Gentle postnatal exercises are suitable for the first six weeks after you have had your baby. After that, provided you have recovered, you should be ready for something a little more energetic. Try joining an exercise class – it's fun exercising with others, and having to go to a class can help sustain flagging motivation. Alternatively, take advantage of the wide range of excellent books and cassettes of postnatal exercises on the market.

unfamiliar people, away from your family and friends. It's not surprising if your emotions are in turmoil. Only if the depression is especially marked or doesn't go away do you need to consult your midwife or doctor (see page 188).

BACK HOME

You may have mixed feelings about going home with your new baby. You're looking forward to taking him home and to looking after him yourself, but you're also worried about how you will cope away from the sanctuary of the hospital. There seems to be such a lot to learn and you can't imagine that you'll ever manage with the cool aplomb of more experienced mothers.

Your baby

Although your baby may seem to have settled into a routine while he was in hospital, once you get him home he seems unpredictable and unsettled. He wants to feed at all hours of the day and night, and the rest of your time is taken up with changing, cleaning, washing and caring for him. Before you had a baby you may have wondered how you would manage to fill the day with only a baby for company. Now you wonder how anyone with children ever has any time for themselves.

In addition, your emotions may be unstable. Rest assured that life does become easier and more predictable. It's normal at first to feel confused and disorganized. After the first six weeks your baby will become more settled and you'll be more used to coping with him. And one magic day, you'll even find he's developed his own routine.

In the meantime, the way to cope is to simplify your life as much as you can.

Coping with tiredness

All new mothers feel tired at first. This tiredness is not just due to physical exhaustion, though this plays a part. Your body needs time to recover from pregnancy and birth, and if you have to get up during the night for feeding it is not surprising that you feel exhausted. You are also mentally tired. You have to take total responsibility 24 hours a day for your new baby. You are probably unsure about how best to look after him, and worried about whether he is getting enough milk, whether he is crying more than he should, whether he is getting enough sleep and so on. With today's small families, most women have not had much contact with a newborn baby before they have their own, so have not acquired the skills and knowledge to make it easy. Preparation can help, and information about what to expect, but it isn't easy. Rest assured that as you become more familiar with your baby and develop your own daily routines the tiredness will pass. Meanwhile try some of the following to help you cope:

- Cut down on all but essential housework.
- Keep meals simple.
- Rest during the day. When your baby is sleeping put your feet up rather than trying to catch up on housework.
- Relax when you give feeds.
- Make sure you have a healthy diet, with plenty of fresh fruit and vegetables. To save time and energy, use tinned or frozen food as the mainstay of your meal, supplemented by a salad and fresh fruit instead of pudding.
- If you are breast-feeding have an extra sandwich or snack to keep up your energy.
- Try to go out at least once a day: walk in the fresh air, breathing deeply.
- Don't skip meals.
- Try to make time to exercise. Just 10 minutes morning and evening will invigorate you. Don't exercise when you are feeling exhausted.
- Practise relaxation, or yoga – there are several good books available on the subject – and 15 minutes' calm relaxation once a day is immensely reviving.
- Take up all offers of help. If you can afford a home help, or are eligible for a local authority one, avail yourself of this until you are feeling stronger.
- Make time for yourself. All work and no play will make you very dull indeed. Go for a walk, read a book, visit the library or friends, or whatever you enjoy doing. Get a babysitter and go out with your partner at least once a week.
- Constant extreme exhaustion can be a first sign of depression. If you feel like this don't struggle on alone, but ask for help from your health visitor or doctor.
- If, despite all this, you still feel physically exhausted, see the doctor

in case you are anaemic. A simple blood test will confirm diagnosis and it can be easily put right by a course of iron treatment.

Visitors

Naturally, all your friends and relatives will want to come and greet the new arrival. However, much as you're glad to see visitors, entertaining them can be tiring. Those who have children themselves are usually aware of this, but others may need a tactful reminder if they are outstaying their welcome. Try to keep visits short – half an hour at the longest – and let your guests help themselves to tea and biscuits. Enlist your husband's help in rationing visitors or tactfully getting rid of those who have stayed too long.

If you are busy bathing the baby or feeding and it's inconvenient to receive guests don't be afraid to ask them politely to call round at another time. You'll be more pleased to see them and a better hostess if you are feeling calm and rested.

Relatives who come to stay can be more problematic. Some relatives are a tremendous help at this time. But if your relatives are not the type to lend a willing hand perhaps they could stay at a guest house or a friend's house. Your baby's and your needs must come first. Even if they do stay in your home try not to make it a long visit. The time for this is when your baby is older and you've settled down to being new parents.

Your midwife and health visitor

The midwife will call on you every day for the first 10 days after your baby's birth. In some areas she will also call once a week for the first month. She is there to check that you are recovering from the birth and to help with any practical problems you may have.

After this period you will be attended by the health visitor, who will be a valued friend in the early years of parenthood. She's a trained nurse (and maybe midwife) who has specialized in the care of babies, young children and their families. She may be attached to your doctor's surgery or a local child health clinic. She's the person to turn to if you want to know anything about your baby's health and welfare. She will give you advice about your baby's immunizations and general health and development checks.

You can visit her at your local child health clinic or your doctor's well-baby clinic (if there is one), where you can have your baby weighed and discuss any problems you may have. If you are at all worried about your baby at any time don't hesitate to contact her – for instance, if you are worried that your baby is ill she can help you decide whether to call the doctor.

She can help you sort out any formal or practical matters too, such as claiming state benefits, finding a child minder, or contacting any community groups in your area. If you have any personal problems, from money worries to sexual difficulties, she'll offer help with those too.

Your health visitor is not there to judge you or the standards of your housekeeping – she is there to help you, so make the most of her!

ESTABLISHING A ROUTINE

New babies are said to sleep an average of 16 to 18 hours a day. If most of your baby's hours of wakefulness are during the evening, or when you would normally be asleep, it can seem that he is awake the whole 24 hours. Life does get easier eventually. In the meantime, be prepared to be flexible and to alter your routine to suit your baby. That way you'll feel less stressed – and a calm mother makes for a calmer baby.

Occasionally you'll need to adjust your baby's routine to fit in with you, for instance when you have to go out or collect your other children from school. In these cases, you can bring the baby's feed forward so that he doesn't start yelling while you are away.

If life seems a complete shambles it may help to write down what you

---

10 tips to help you cope

- Cut down on your social life until your baby is more settled.
- Bear in mind that the first few weeks are the most difficult.
- Keep one room tidy for entertaining visitors.
- Don't be in too much of a hurry to get your baby into a routine.
- Share your feelings with your husband.
- If you miss the company of your workmates find out about postnatal groups in your area – your health visitor will be able to give you details.
- Discuss any practical problems you may have, such as money worries.
- Make time for your husband, even if it's only short. Sit down over a meal together or watch television.
- Keep your postnatal check-up appointment so any physical problems can be sorted out.
- Learn how to manage disagreements. It may be a matter of compromising, or of taking turns.

have to do in the day. Then, after the first few weeks, you can keep a note of the times of day when your baby usually sleeps, feeds, and so on. With these records you can plan to fit in the tasks you have to do. Don't be too ambitious, though, otherwise you won't fit everything in and you'll feel frustrated. Try to stick to one major project each day, such as the ironing or the shopping, but don't become too rigid about it. There are bound to be days when your baby simply won't settle, and you'll both become tired and irritable if you insist on following your plan.

Enjoy your baby

A new baby needs four things – food, drink, warmth and love. If you can provide him with all these you are doing a good job. If your baby sleeps reasonably well, takes his food, and produces six or more wet nappies a day and soft yellow bowel motions you can be sure he is thriving physically.

Some babies cry more than others – if he had a difficult birth he may be more irritable and difficult to calm in the first few weeks. Some babies seem more jumpy and nervous by nature. Research has shown that babies who have their cries for attention dealt with promptly cry less in the long term than babies who are left to cry long and hard before anyone responds to them. It stands to reason if you think about it.

> *Why is my baby crying?*
>
> Babies cry for lots of reasons. As he gets older you'll get more skilful at interpreting his cries. In the meantime, these are some of the most common causes:
>
> - Hunger
> - Wind or colic
> - Soreness or discomfort
> - Tiredness
> - Overstimulation
> - Fear
> - Loneliness
>
> You'll find out by trial and error the best way to comfort your baby. Some tried-and-tested remedies include wrapping him firmly in a shawl or blanket, vigorous rocking, singing, or walking up and down with him.
>
> More information on the causes of crying and how to cope appears in *The Mother and Baby Book of Your Baby's First Year*.

The secret of successful parenting is to stay calm and not expect too much of yourself or your baby. If you can learn to relax about it and realize that everyone makes mistakes from time to time, you'll enjoy it a lot more.

There's no such thing as a perfect parent – and most children grow up to be reasonably well-balanced adults despite their parents! The child psychologist Donald Winnicott coined the term 'good enough' parenting to describe the happy medium we should aim for. It can help to bear this in mind if you're tempted to be too hard on yourself.

You and your husband – now that you're parents

The arrival of a new baby is often presented as a sure-fire way of living happily ever after – but there are many adjustments you both have to make.

The reality of a new baby, who seems to want feeding all the time and never seems to sleep, can put strains on your relationship. There are other stresses too. As the mother, being at home all day is probably an unfamiliar experience – you may miss your wage packet and the company of your workmates. What's more, looking after a baby is different in nature from any other sort of job. Baby care involves a seemingly endless round of the same chores – which never seem to be finished.

For the first time in your life you and your husband occupy separate worlds. He is out at work all day and you are at home. He may feel under pressure to take on overtime, or he may worry about his ability to provide for his new family.

Meanwhile, at the very time you feel the need to be cared for and supported everything revolves around the baby. And, with all the physical and emotional changes going on in your life, you may not feel much like sex.

It's hardly surprising that the birth of a baby is such a turning point for couples. Appreciating the emotions you are each experiencing helps to ease any strain, and with plenty of give and take you and your husband can become closer, even though your relationship is changed.

WHEN WILL I FEEL LIKE MAKING LOVE AGAIN?

Some women feel ready to make love almost as soon as they have had their babies. However, it's perfectly normal and common to lose interest in sex for as long as several months after having a baby, especially if stitches are making you uncomfortable.

Breast-feeding makes some women feel especially sexy, but others don't feel a return of desire until after they have stopped feeding.

Sometimes birth can activate either partner's long-standing, underlying anxieties about sex. If you feel there is a real problem it will help to talk to your doctor or a marriage guidance counsellor. Don't feel embarrassed – they are not easily shocked, and many couples have been helped by such counselling.

Even if you don't feel like intercourse there are plenty of ways of showing your affection for each other, such as massage, stroking, and mutual masturbation.

When you start to make love again, you may feel a bit nervous. Take your time, and make sure your baby is first fed and settled so that you're not interrupted.

The natural lubrication of the vagina sometimes doesn't return for several weeks, so it is advisable to use a lubricant such as KY jelly. Your husband should wait until you are fully aroused before entering you. You may feel more comfortable, and if you are breast-feeding there will be less pressure on your breasts, if you are on top of him. This way you will be able to control the depth of penetration. You may find, if you are breast-feeding, that milk spurts from your nipples as you reach a climax. It's less likely to happen if your breasts are empty, which is another good reason to feed the baby before you start love-making. Simply protect the sheet with a towel.

Making love again

- Make love when you feel ready – not before.
- Use plenty of lubrication and relax your pelvic floor muscles as your husband penetrates you.
- Use pillows under your pelvis to take any pressure off scarred areas.
- Don't assume you must always make love at night, when you may feel tired and disinclined. If the baby is asleep, take the phone off the hook, draw the curtains and make the most of it.
- Keep a sense of humour if things aren't successful for the first few times.
- Use a reliable contraceptive (see page 186).

Your postnatal check-up

You will be given an appointment for your postnatal check-up when you leave hospital or when you are signed off by your doctor or midwife. It's important to keep this appointment, so that any problems you might have can be resolved at an early stage. If you can't keep the appointment, make another one.

Try to have your baby looked after when you go for the check-up. You'll be more relaxed than if you're listening for the sound of your baby's crying.

What will happen?

The postnatal is rather like an antenatal, except that the doctor is looking for signs that your body has returned to normal.

You'll be weighed, your blood pressure, blood and urine will be tested and you'll have an internal examination to check that your vagina and pelvic organs have returned to normal. The doctor will gently feel your perineum to check that any stitches have healed properly. He or she will feel your abdomen to make sure that your uterus has contracted to its usual size, and gently probe the top of your vagina and ovaries to make sure they are not swollen, abnormal or tender.

If you want to slim you will be given advice on dieting. Any signs of anaemia will be dealt with by a course of iron tablets or vitamins. If you were not immune to rubella (German measles) before your pregnancy and you received no immunization in hospital you'll now be given the vaccination.

An opportunity to discuss any problems

There will be the opportunity to discuss your pregnancy and delivery. If there were any complications during birth your doctor will explain what happened and why, and will give you some idea of whether they will occur again. If you have any problems with breast-feeding, periods, backache or sexual worries, now is the time to raise them. If your baby was abnormal in any way, you are probably worried in case it happens again. Spend some time talking to the doctor about your feelings. If the problem is an inherited one, your doctor will be able to refer you for genetic counselling. An expert who has studied the patterns of disease in families will take full details of your family tree and will be able to work out the probability of the same thing happening again. If there is a high risk of the same problem occurring, you will be offered special screening during your next pregnancy, so that if you wish, the pregnancy may be terminated.

CONTRACEPTION

As soon as you start having intercourse again you will need to use contraception in order to avoid becoming pregnant. If you are breast-feeding, your periods will probably be delayed until you start the baby on solids, or even wean her completely. However, ovulation (the production of an egg) takes place a couple of weeks before you have your period, and conception can take place. Complete breast-feeding on demand usually reduces fertility but is not entirely reliable as a contraceptive. If you are bottle-feeding, menstruation can occur after four to six weeks.

You can get advice on contraception from your family doctor or the family planning clinic. Alternatively the doctor at your postnatal check-up may advise you and fit you with an IUD or cap if this is your choice, providing, of course, you have recovered internally. You may want to change the type of contraception you use either temporarily or permanently now you have had a baby. The Family Planning Association has written a number of useful leaflets, which are available in family planning clinics and doctors' surgeries, to help you decide which is the most suitable form of contraception for you.

You may find that a combination of methods suits you best, but whatever type of contraception you choose, do follow the instructions exactly. Unless you intend to get pregnant again straight away, worrying about becoming pregnant can mar your enjoyment of your baby.

The condom (sheath)
This is a useful and reliable method of contraception when properly used. The only disadvantage is that after you have had a baby your vagina may be temporarily insufficiently lubricated, or still feeling sore as a result of an episiotomy. The solution is to use a lubricant such as KY jelly or a spermicidal cream or foam in conjunction with the condom. These can be obtained from a family planning clinic or your doctor. Alternatively you can buy them over the counter at a chemist's.

The pill

If you are breast-feeding you may dislike the thought of taking a hormone which can pass through the milk to your baby. The combined pill, which contains the hormones oestrogen and progesterone, is unsuitable anyway. It can affect the quantity and quality of your milk supply, and induces subtle changes in your body. No one knows whether there are any long-term harmful effects on the baby. The low-dose progesterone-only pill, sometimes known as the mini-pill, is the one most commonly prescribed for breast-feeding mothers, since only minimal doses of the hormone are used. It works by thickening the cervical mucus, so making it hostile to sperm, rather than by preventing ovulation as the combined pill does.

However, this means it is slightly less effective, and you should make especially sure you take the pill at exactly the same time every day. A course of antibiotics or an episode of diarrhoea or vomiting can cancel out the contraceptive effect, and in order to avoid pregnancy you should use another method of contraception until you start the next course of pills.

Intrauterine device (IUD)

This is an extremely reliable form of contraception. It is easier to insert once you have had a baby because the cervix is slightly stretched and your uterus is less likely to reject it. No one knows how it works, but it may be by causing certain chemical changes in the uterus to prevent the sperm from fusing with the egg. The IUD has no effect on the baby, and avoids the more mechanical aspects of the barrier methods (condom and cap) which some couples find offputting. The main disadvantage is that there is an increased risk of pelvic infection.

Natural fertility control

As methods of contraception such as the pill and IUD come under increased suspicion of causing health problems, many couples are turning to natural family planning techniques, which involve awareness of the female cycle. The method relies on techniques such as daily temperature-taking, and observing the cervical mucus, which changes in nature over the course of the menstrual cycle. If taught and used correctly, natural fertility control can be both safe and effective. However, after childbirth and during breast-feeding, because the hormone balance of your body has not returned to normal, it may be

best to combine the method with barrier techniques for greater
reliability. Be guided by your medical adviser or natural fertility
teacher.

Diaphragm (cap)
If you were using one of these before having your baby, you will need to
have a new one fitted because your internal dimensions will have
changed. The doctor will be able to do this accurately about six weeks
after childbirth. If the vaginal muscles are still slack following birth,
the spring-rim type of cap may not be suitable, since it relies on muscle
tone to hold it in place. In this case you can change to a cervical cap,
which fits snugly over the cervix. You will need to use a spermicide
with this method of contraception for greater reliability.

Collagen sponge
This is a sponge impregnated with spermicide, which is said to be
around 75 per cent effective. However, it may be less effective when
your vagina has been stretched as a result of birth. If you definitely
don't want to become pregnant it is probably advisable to use another
method.

Coitus interruptus (withdrawal)
This technique, which relies on the man withdrawing his penis from
the vagina before ejaculating, is not reliable. It demands great control
on the man's part, and sperm may be released in the fluid that is present
before ejaculation. Furthermore, sperm can swim up from the outside of
the vagina to the uterus.

IF THE BLUES DON'T GO AWAY

Most new mothers are slightly emotionally unstable during the weeks
following birth. It's only natural considering the revolution a baby
causes, physically and in many other ways. However, if you continue to
feel tired, weepy, and lacking all interest in life you could be suffering
from the more serious condition of postnatal depression.

Postnatal depression may be mild or severe. It can emerge a few
weeks to a few months after your baby's birth and may last for weeks or
months. In fact, despite its name, depression may not be the main

> ### POSTNATAL DEPRESSION – HOW YOU CAN HELP YOURSELF
>
> *Before the birth*
>
> - Find out about local mothers' groups in your area by asking your midwife or visiting the local library or citizen's advice bureau.
> - Try to make friends with someone who already has a baby or children.
> - Find out as much as you can about babies by reading magazines such as *Mother & Baby*, talking with people who have children, and so on.
> - Talk with your partner about some of the adjustments you will have to make after the birth. Work out practical strategies for dealing with some of these changes.
>
> *After the birth*
>
> - Follow a good diet with plenty of wholefoods, and eat foods rich in vitamin B (see chart on page 60).
> - Build rest and relaxation into your daily routine.
> - Make time to do something for yourself.
> - Get out and about with the baby.
> - If you become depressed don't keep it to yourself.

symptom at all – anxiety, insomnia, irritability, lack of appetite and the feeling that life is too much for you, can all be symptoms.

The good news is that it can be treated. So if you experience any of these symptoms contact your health visitor or doctor without delay. The sooner you get help the sooner you'll start to feel better.

Some sufferers benefit from anti-depressant drugs or vitamin B6 and B3. For others extra help, practical support and counselling can relieve the condition. Depression may be a useful pointer to you to have the extra rest and care that you need. Talking about your fears and worries with, perhaps, your health visitor, a close friend or a former sufferer, can be one of the most valuable forms of treatment.

Will I get postnatal depression?

Recent research has indicated that some women are especially vulnerable to postnatal depression. These include:

- Those who have previously had mental or emotional problems, including a former bout of postnatal depression.
- Those who don't have a close relationship with their husband.
- Those who don't have close friends or confidants.

- Those who find change of any sort difficult and anxiety-provoking.
- Those who have experienced a particularly difficult labour, delay, caesarean, forceps, and so on.

BECOMING PARENTS

The birth of a new human being is always cause for celebration. It is also frequently a time for reflection: for looking back to the past and forward towards the future. Whether this has been your first or a subsequent baby, the addition of this new person to your life will change it irrevocably. Especially if this is your first child, you will have had much to absorb and come to terms with over the last few months. In just under the course of a year you and your husband have changed from being a couple to being parents. And whether this was planned or an unanticipated pregnancy, it will have changed the way you think about yourself. For the first time in your life you may be feeling truly 'grown-up'. Yet at the same time you may feel totally unsure of yourself. The birth of any child, but especially a first one, often brings both feelings of loss and gain: loss of your former identity, even of the baby you imagined you would have; gain of a new role, and the baby you are beginning to get to know. Such mixed feelings are quite normal. As with all major adjustments in life it can take a while before you feel entirely secure in your new role.

In this book we have dealt with many of the problems and anxieties that beset couples as they go through the process of becoming parents. We hope that the information contained has helped to allay fears and worries, so that you have been able to enjoy the transition – at least some of the time.

Once you have your baby new preoccupations surface – feeding, nappies, sleeping habits. But these practical anxieties often mask deeper questions about your new role as a parent: 'Can I cope?' 'Will I be good enough?' It is reassuring to realize that although the details of your child's needs will change with her growing maturity, her underlying needs are basically the same. Above all, she wants and needs your love and affection, and your pride in her as a worthwhile human being. That means not just catering for her physical well-being, but being alert to her emotional and mental needs. Fortunately this need not be burdensome. Your child is born with an overwhelming curiosity to find out about the world in which she lives. So long as you provide her with a safe environment in which to explore, this inbuilt urge to know will take care of the rest. Of course, there are many ways in which you can encourage her desire for knowledge, by providing her with new experiences, toys, games, and so on to foster her growing abilities and skills. But more than any of these your child needs you to be there for her, and to show that you appreciate her as the unique individual she is, and not the person you think she should be.

At first your baby is egocentric: she believes the world revolves around her and her needs. As she gets bigger and more aware she begins to recognize how her actions affect others around her, and in turn how their actions affect her. The skills she learns in her relationships with members of her family prepare and equip her for the task of relating to others in the outside world.

Of course you and your husband have needs too. There is no reason to be swamped by the demands of parenthood. With careful management you should be able to take some time off to pursue your own interests and to develop as a person. In fact you will be a better parent if you do not neglect your own needs. Once the first few demanding months of parenthood are past, make the effort to organize some time to yourself once in a while. You will come back to your job of parenting with renewed vitality.

WHAT KIND OF PARENTS WILL WE BE?

Your style of parenting will be influenced by many factors: how you and your husband were brought up yourselves, the ideas you have developed since then, the people you mix with, what you have read, and, last but not least, your interaction with your child. The combination of these will result in your own unique way of bringing up a child.

There is no one right way to raise a child. So long as your child develops into a happy individual who is able to enjoy life to the full, you will have done a good job. You may admire the way your own parents brought you up, and want to emulate it, or you may reject some of the values they brought you up to believe in. The same goes for your husband. Most probably you will want to retain some aspects of your own upbringing and discard others. Even so it's not always easy to change; you may find yourself behaving in the same way as your own mother and father – without realizing how or why. It helps to talk to each other about the sorts of messages, both overt and hidden, you picked up from your own childhood, and the expectations you have of yourself and each other as parents. Bringing these things into the open will help you to make conscious decisions about the ways in which you would like to bring up *your* child, and can alleviate conflict.

Our parents are the models on whom, often unconsciously, we have based ourselves, and these models often surface only when we become parents ourselves. It can be hard to break old patterns, even when you intend to. You and your husband may be quite happy with the traditional division of labour, in which the man's main responsibility is to be the breadwinner, and the woman's is to look after home and family. An increasingly common pattern nowadays is for parents to divide up the tasks of earning, childcare and housework more equally. But, despite one or two well-publicized examples, complete role reversals, in which the woman goes out to work to support the family and the man stays at home, are still relatively rare, partly because most women's earning power is still lower than men's. Another change in family life over the last decade has been the growing number of single parents who are bringing up a child alone, either through choice or necessity. It helps to realize that no one type of family set-up has been shown to be better than any other for raising children. Children throughout the ages and in different parts of the world have survived and flourished in a wide diversity of family groups. Whether you are bringing up your child in the traditional nuclear group, as part of a large extended family of grandparents, aunts, uncles and other relatives, or as a lone parent, or in any other type of household, your child needs to know that you love and appreciate her. Safe in this knowledge she stands an excellent chance of growing up to be a secure, happy individual, whatever her background.

OTHER PEOPLE

One of the unexpected bonuses of parenthood is the bond that it forges between people of different generations, races and beliefs. Babies break down barriers in a way that it is difficult to imagine before you have children. Many a lifelong friendship has been forged in the first hazy moments on the postnatal ward. It's a process that continues as your child grows up and comes into contact with the outside world. The others you meet at toddler group, in the cluster around the school gate, at sports' days or in connection with your child's hobbies, can support you as you journey through the pleasures and anxieties of parenthood together.

YOUR CHILD

At the centre of it all is your child. What you make of parenthood depends almost as much on her as on you. Each child is a unique individual with her own personality and way of relating to others. As you watch your baby grow from a tiny dependent being into a boisterous toddler and then an independent, lively young person, you will be shaped by her and her way of looking at things. Parents have as much to learn from their children as children have to learn from them, and this is what makes the whole experience so fascinating. Most parents agree that, despite the sacrifices it generally involves, bringing up children is one of the most rewarding activities they have ever undertaken.

There will be times when the burden seems overwhelming, and you won't always get things 'right'. Try not to expect too much of yourself, and concentrate on the things you *are* doing well. You can't be perfect and all parents make mistakes. But as your child grows, you and your husband will come to know yourselves better too. You will discover strengths and resources that you didn't know you possessed. Don't try to bury the problems, but don't dwell on them to the exclusion of all the good things either. Cherish those happy moments when your baby slips off the breast like a sleepy bee, admire her velvety skin and her downy head, feel proud of her first smile. There will be many more such experiences to come. Enjoy them!

Glossary

Abdomen. The lower part of the stomach that contains your uterus.

Abruptio placenta. See Placental abruption.

Acceleration. The process of augmenting contractions by means of a hormone drip, in order to speed up labour or make contractions more effective.

Alpha-feto-protein (AFP). A substance produced by the baby which is detectable in your blood stream. A test to measure AFP level is performed at around 12 weeks of pregnancy, as high levels can indicate problems such as spina bifida, Down's syndrome, or a twin pregnancy.

Amniocentesis. A test that involves drawing off a sample of the amniotic fluid surrounding the baby in order to detect abnormalities or the sex of the baby. In later pregnancy it can be used to assess maturity of the lungs.

Amniotic fluid. Also known as liquor, the waters in which your baby floats during pregnancy.

Anaemia. Lack of haemoglobin in the red blood cells.

Anaesthetic. Medication producing pain relief, e.g. epidural. A local anaesthetic affects only part of the body. A complete anaesthetic affects the whole body and usually means loss of consciousness. You may need one if you have a caesarean.

Analgesic. Pain-killing agent.

Antenatal. Before the birth.

Anterior presentation. Refers to the way the baby is lying in the uterus. The anterior is the most usual presentation, in which the baby's body is towards your backbone.

Apgar test or score. A standard test used to check the baby's condition immediately after birth.

Areola. The pigmented area around the nipple.

ARM (Artificial Rupture of the Membranes). The surgical rupture of the bag of waters in which your baby is floating (amniotic sac). Also called amniotomy. It is often used to induce labour in combination with drugs to start the uterus contracting.

Bearing down. The massive urge to push down into the birth canal in the second stage of labour.

Bilirubin. Broken-down red blood cells which are normally cleared by the liver. If the level is too high, jaundice occurs. A high bilirubin level in the amniotic fluid is an indication of Rhesus problems.

Braxton-Hicks contractions. Painless tightenings of the uterus which occur throughout pregnancy, often without you noticing them. They help maintain vigorous circulation to the uterus and aid its growth.

Breech presentation. The position of a baby who is lying bottom down in the uterus. The legs or the bottom may be born first.

Brow presentation. When the baby is lying head down but with the brow placed so that it will come through the cervix first. Often an indication for a caesarean, as the brow is the widest part.

GLOSSARY

Butterfly mask. Mild pigmentation of face during pregnancy. Otherwise known as chloasma or mask of pregnancy.

Caesarean section. The delivery of the baby by means of a surgical incision through the abdomen and uterus.

Carpal tunnel syndrome. Fluid build-up in the wrists which presses on the nerves, causing tingling and numbness.

Catheter. A thin, fine tube inserted into the body; for example it may be inserted into the tube leading from your bladder to draw off urine, or the epidural space to drip in anaesthetic.

Cephalic presentation. The position of the baby who is lying head down in the uterus.

Cervix. The neck of the womb or uterus.

Chorionic gonadotrophin. See HCG.

Chorionic villus sampling (CVS). A test which involves taking a sample of the developing placenta. It gives information on certain hereditary and chromosome disorders, as well as the sex of the baby.

Colostrum. The fluid produced in the breasts during pregnancy and the first few days after birth. It contains concentrated nutrients and antibodies.

Community midwife. A midwife who is based outside the hospital. She will deliver you if you have your baby at home or if you have a domino delivery, and will visit you daily at home when you are discharged from hospital.

Complementary feed. A top-up bottle-feed given in addition to the breast.

Contractions. The regular tightening of the muscles of the uterus during labour.

Co-operation card. The card on which all the important medical details about your pregnancy are recorded.

Crowning. The moment during delivery when the baby's head appears in the vagina.

Dehydration. Loss of bodily fluid.

Demand feeding. Feeding the baby whenever he is hungry rather than according to the clock.

Diabetes. A condition in which the body fails to metabolize sugar. It can sometimes appear during pregnancy and disappear after childbirth. This is called gestational diabetes. Sugar in the urine can be an indication of diabetes, and is one of the things tested for when your urine is tested at the antenatal clinic.

Diaphragm. The dome-shaped muscles separating the chest cavity from the abdomen.

Diaphragm (contraceptive cap). A type of contraception that works by blocking the cervix to prevent sperm swimming into it.

Dilatation. The process by which the cervix opens up during labour.

Disproportion. When there is lack of fit between the baby's head and the mother's pelvis, leading to a caesarean section.

Domino scheme. A service operated by community midwives, who look after you antenatally, take you into hospital when labour starts, deliver the baby, and then accompany you home. It stands for Domiciliary-in-out.

Doppler ultrasound. A type of scan which measures the flow of blood in the placenta and the baby's blood vessels.

Down's syndrome. A chromosomal disorder most common in babies born to mothers in their late thirties and beyond. It used to be known as mongolism.

Drip. The procedure which allows fluid, e.g. sugar or a drug, to be fed directly into the blood stream by means of a thin tube which is introduced into a vein. Labour is often induced or accelerated by means of a drip containing oxytocin.

Ectopic pregnancy. When the fertilized egg embeds in the fallopian tube rather than the uterus. The pregnancy usually ends around the 10th week. Symptoms are severe pain, vomiting and faintness.

EDD. Expected or estimated date of delivery. The date on which your baby is due. This is only approximate, though most babies are born within two weeks on either side of the EDD.

Electronic fetal monitoring (EFM). The monitoring of the baby's heart beat by means of a transducer placed on your abdomen, or an electrode which is clipped or screwed to the baby's scalp.

Embryo. The developing baby from the 10th day after fertilization to the 12th week of pregnancy.

Enema. The insertion of the contents of a small bag of salted water into the rectum to induce a bowel motion. Sometimes given as part of the preparation procedure when you go into the labour ward.

Engagement of the head. When the head drops down into the pelvis towards the end of pregnancy in preparation for birth. In a first pregnancy this can happen from about the 37th week. In a second or subsequent one, it may not engage until just before or during labour. It is popularly known as lightening.

Engorgement. The temporary swelling of the breasts that occurs during the first week of breast-feeding, caused by increased blood supply to the breasts plus the beginning of milk production.

Entonox. The brand name given to the mixture of nitrous oxide and oxygen (gas and air) which is inhaled for pain relief during the first stage of labour.

Epidural. A type of anaesthetic used for labour and for caesarean sections, in which an anaesthetic is injected into a space in the lower spine.

Episiotomy. A cut made in the perineum (skin between the vagina and the anus) just before the baby is born.

Expressing milk. The drawing off of breast milk by hand or pump.

Face presentation. The position in which the baby's face is the first part to be born.

Fallopian tubes. The two narrow tubes that lead from the uterus to the ovary.

False labour. Strong Braxton-Hicks contractions that are confused with the longer, stronger, more regular contractions of true labour.

Fertilization. The meeting of the sperm and the ovum (egg) to create an embryo.

Fetal distress. The condition in which the fetus is short of oxygen during labour or late pregnancy. Signs are changes in the heart rate and the presence of meconium in the amniotic fluid.

Fetal movements. Known popularly as quickening. The movements of the baby in the womb, which can be felt from about the 20th week onwards.

Fetoscope. A fine tube which is inserted into the uterus in order to photograph the fetus to check for abnormalities.

GLOSSARY

Fetus. The developing baby in the uterus from the 12th week of pregnancy until birth.

Folic acid. A B vitamin which is especially important in pregnancy for the formation of red blood cells and the absorption of iron.

Forceps. Instruments used to help the baby out of the birth canal when either the baby or the mother is too ill or too tired to continue with normal labour. They are usually shaped like a pair of hinged spoons.

Fundus. The top of the uterus.

Gas and air. See Entonox.

Gene. The part of the cell which contains each individual's hereditary blueprint, e.g. blood group, height, eye colour and so on.

Genetic counselling. The process of being advised by a specialist in medical genetics about the likelihood of passing on an inherited disease or condition to your children.

Glucose. A natural sugar which is the main source of energy. A glucose drip is sometimes set up during labour if you are running short of energy.

GP Unit. General practitioner unit. This may be a small hospital delivering babies under the supervision of local GPs or a unit within the main maternity unit. Intended for women expecting normal deliveries.

Gynaecologist. A doctor specializing in female illnesses and conditions.

Haemoglobin. A compound in the red blood cells. Anaemia shows up as a low haemoglobin level.

Haemorrhage. A bleed, in pregnancy or after birth, from the site of the placenta.

HCG. Human chorionic gonadotrophin, a hormone secreted by the fertilized egg. This is the substance looked for in pregnancy tests, as it is found in the pregnant woman's urine from seven days after a missed period.

Hypertension. High blood pressure.

Hypotension. Low blood pressure.

Implantation. The embedding of the fertilized egg in the uterus.

Incompetent cervix. A cervix which won't remain closed during pregnancy, leading to late miscarriage. Once diagnosed, a special stitch can be inserted to hold it closed until just before the baby's birth.

Induction. The process of starting off labour artificially.

Internal monitoring. See electronic fetal monitoring.

Intravenous drip. See Drip.

Inverted nipples. Nipples that turn inwards rather than protruding.

Involution of the uterus. The process by which the uterus returns to the non-pregnant state after childbirth.

Iron. An essential mineral necessary for haemoglobin production.

Jaundice. The yellowish tinge of the skin sometimes seen in newborn babies as a result of their livers being too immature to cope with the breakdown of red blood cells.

Ketones. Substances that appear in the urine when the body's carbohydrate stores are depleted. If ketones appear in the urine during labour body chemistry is disturbed and labour can slow down. The most usual solution is to set up a glucose drip.

Kick chart. A chart on which the baby's movements are recorded, so as to indicate his well-being.

Labour. The birth process. It is divided into three stages: in the first stage the cervix opens up (dilates); in the second stage the baby is pushed down the birth canal; and in the third stage the placenta is delivered.

Lateral position. When the baby is lying across the uterus. Also known as transverse position. If the baby is in this position at the onset of labour a caesarean is necessary.

Let-down reflex. The hormone reflex responsible for ejecting milk from the nipple. It is caused by the hormone oxytocin.

LH. Luteinizing hormone. A hormone secreted by the pituitary gland at ovulation. A surge of this can indicate your most fertile period, and is the basis for modern fertility tests.

Lie of baby. The way the baby is lying in the uterus.

Lightening. See Engagement.

Linea nigra. A dark line of pigment from the navel to the pubis that appears during pregnancy.

Lithotomy position. The position in which the mother lies flat on her back with her legs raised and bent at the knees, and supported in stirrups. A common delivery position which has been widely criticized on the grounds that it is unphysiological.

Lochia. A discharge that comes from the uterus in the weeks after birth.

Meconium. The first substance to be passed from your baby's bowels. It is thick, sticky and greenish black in colour. The presence of meconium in the amniotic fluid (waters) during pregnancy or birth is a sign of fetal distress.

Membranes. The tissues that contain the baby and the amniotic fluid in the uterus. Popularly known as the bag of waters.

Miscarriage. The loss of a baby before 28 weeks' gestation. Known medically as an abortion.

Montgomery's tubercles. The small bumps on the areola that appear in pregnancy. They secrete a lubricating fluid to keep the skin soft.

Multiple pregnancy. When you are carrying more than one baby.

NAD. Medical term meaning nothing abnormal detected. You can expect to see it on your co-operation card.

Natural childbirth. A childbirth that proceeds without medical help or intervention, especially in the form of drugs or machinery.

Nausea. The sick feeling that is especially common in the first three months of pregnancy.

Navel. Otherwise known as the umbilicus, the site of the umbilical cord in the middle of the abdomen.

Occipito posterior. The position in which the baby's back is towards your back, either to the right or the left. When the baby is in this position labour tends to be longer and more uncomfortable.

Occiput. The back of the baby's head.

Oedema. Fluid retention. It can be a sign of pre-eclampsia.

Oestriol. A hormone secreted by the placenta. It can be tested for in the urine and blood in late pregnancy to see how well the placenta is functioning.

GLOSSARY

Operculum. The medical name for the 'show' or plug of mucus that seals the cervix during pregnancy.

Os of the cervix. The opening of the cervix.

Oxytocin. A hormone produced by the pituitary gland which causes the uterus to contract. A synthetic form of the hormone is used in a drip to induce or accelerate labour. It is the hormone involved in the let-down reflex.

Palpation. Feeling the parts of the baby inside the uterus, by pressing gently on the abdomen.

Partogram. A chart used to record the progress of labour and the baby's condition.

Pelvic floor. The sheets of muscle which support the pelvic organs.

Perinatal. The time from just before delivery to seven days afterwards. Perinatal death is the death of a baby just before, during or in the week following birth.

Perineum. The area between the vagina and the anus, which is cut when an episiotomy is performed.

Pessaries. Vaginal suppositories. Prostaglandin pessaries are often used to induce labour.

Pethidine. A narcotic (sleep-inducing) drug given to relax the mother during labour.

Placenta. The afterbirth. A gland which attaches itself to the uterus and is linked to the baby by means of the umbilical cord, to supply him with nutrients and oxygen, and pass back his waste products into the mother's blood system.

Placental abruption (abruptio placenta). When the placenta starts to peel away from the uterus in late pregnancy, causing bleeding and sometimes pain.

Placental insufficiency. A condition in which the placenta is failing to function properly so that the baby does not grow as he should.

Placenta praevia. A condition in which the placenta is lying low down in the uterus, sometimes partially or wholly blocking the outlet.

Posterior position. See Occipito posterior.

Postnatal. After the birth, as in postnatal depression: a depressed state that can include feelings of sadness, exhaustion, anxiety, inability to cope, and so on.

Postnatal examination. The medical check-up that takes place approximately six weeks after birth to check that your body has returned to normal after pregnancy and childbirth.

Post-partum haemorrhage. A heavy loss of blood after delivery, which can be dangerous unless it is stemmed.

Pre-eclampsia, or pre-eclamptic toxaemia. A high blood pressure condition that occurs during pregnancy, causing the blood vessels of the placenta to shut down. It can be dangerous to the baby, and immediate delivery may be required. Its symptoms are headaches, dizziness and nausea or vomiting, but these do not occur until the illness has become severe.

Prepping. A term used by midwives to describe the preparations you are given for labour when you go into hospital to have the baby. These can include physical examination, taking the baby's heart beat and, less often nowadays, a shave and enema, or breaking the waters.

Preterm baby, or premature baby. A baby born before the 37th week of pregnancy.

Primigravida. A woman who is pregnant for the first time.

Prolapsed cord. A rare complication of labour in which the umbilical cord drops down in front of the baby's head and can become compressed.

Prostaglandins. Natural, hormone-like substances that occur in the body and stimulate the onset of labour. Prostaglandin pessaries or gel are often used to induce labour.

Protein in the urine. Protein detected in the urine during pregnancy can indicate a vaginal or urinary infection, or sometimes pre-eclampsia.

Psychoprophylaxis. Literally meaning mind prevention, this describes a set of breathing and distraction techniques designed to take your mind off the pain of labour. It forms the basis of some antenatal classes.

Puerperium. The time after delivery.

Quickening. The first sensations of the baby's movement in the uterus, usually felt around 20 weeks with a first baby, earlier with subsequent ones.

Recurrent abortion. Repeated miscarriage.

Rhesus factor. An antigen (immunity-producing substance) found in the red blood cells of people who are Rhesus positive.

Rooming in. The practice of keeping mothers and babies next to each other on the postnatal ward, rather than putting the babies in a nursery.

Rubella (German measles). A virus which can harm the baby, causing deafness, blindness or other abnormalities, if contracted during the first three months of pregnancy.

Scan. See Ultrasound scan.

Shared care. A system of antenatal care which is shared between the GP and the hospital.

Show. A discharge of blood-stained mucus from the vagina, caused by the plug of mucus which seals the cervix during pregnancy being expelled as the result of the cervix dilating.

Sickle cell anaemia. A serious form of anaemia found in people of African, Asian, Arab and West Indian origin.

Spina bifida. A congenital condition (i.e. present at birth) in which the spinal cord forms outside the spinal column.

Stillbirth. The delivery of a dead baby after 28 weeks of pregnancy, as the result of abnormality, separation of the placenta, placental insufficiency and some infections.

Stretch marks. Red, spidery lines that appear on the surface of the abdomen, thighs, buttocks and breasts as a result of the tearing of deeper skin layers. After pregnancy they gradually fade to a silvery colour.

Syntocinon. The brand name of synthetic oxytocin, which is used to speed up or induce labour.

TENs or TNS. Transcutaneous electrical nerve stimulation. A method of pain relief which works by transmitting electrical impulses from a battery-operated box in order to block pain messages coming from the uterus.

GLOSSARY

Term. The end of pregnancy. Approximately 40 weeks after the last menstrual period.

Thalassaemia. An inherited type of anaemia found most often in people of Mediterranean and Asian origin.

Thrombosis. A clot of blood in a vein.

Toxaemia. See Pre-eclampsia.

Transducer. An instrument which is sensitive to the echoes of sound waves bounced off the developing baby in the uterus.

Transition. The period between the first and second stage of labour.

Transverse position. See Lateral position.

Trimester. A third of pregnancy. Pregnancy is divided into three trimesters.

Ultrasound scan. A way of studying the baby in the uterus by means of sound waves, which are bounced off his body and converted into an image on a TV screen.

Umbilical cord. The lifeline between your baby and the placenta. It contains two arteries which transport used blood back to the placenta and a vein which carries oxygenated blood to the baby.

Urine test. A test which is carried out during every antenatal visit to check for protein, sugar, signs of infection and ketones.

Uterus. The womb.

Vacuum extraction. A process of helping the baby out of the vagina by means of a suction device called a ventouse. It is an alternative to forceps.

Vagina. The canal that leads from the external genitals to the cervix, down which the baby passes during birth.

VE. Vaginal examination.

Ventouse. A metal or plastic cup attached to a pump. The cup adheres to the baby's head by suction, and can be used to draw the baby gently down the birth canal as an alternative to forceps.

Vernix. The greasy substance produced by the baby's skin which covers him from 30 weeks, and protects his skin from drying out.

X-rays. Electromagnetic waves used to photograph the skeleton. Because of the risk of radiation to the baby, X-rays are done only when strictly necessary during pregnancy, for example because there is thought to be some disproportion, or if the baby is breech.

Useful addresses

The organizations listed below offer support, advice and information. Many have a widespread network of local branches. Contact the addresses below to find your nearest branch. Since many of these organizations are charities they do appreciate an s.a.e.

Antenatal classes
Active Birth Movement, 55 Dartmouth Park Road, London NW5 1SL. Tel: 01-267 3006
National Childbirth Trust, Alexandra House, Oldham Terrace, Acton, London, W3 6NH. Tel: 01-992 8637
Birth Centres, contact the Active Birth Movement (see above) for details.

Pregnancy
Miscarriage Association, 18 Stoneybrook Close, West Bretton, Wakefield, West Yorkshire WF4 4TP. Tel: 0924 85515
Society to Support Home Confinements, Ludgate House, Ludgate Lane, Wolsingham, Bishop Auckland, Durham DL13 3HA. Tel: 0388 528044
ASH (*Action on Smoking and Health*), 5–11 Mortimer Street, London W1N 7RH. Tel: 01-637 9843
TENS equipment is available from Neen Pain Management Systems, Barn Lodge, Gooseberry Hill, Swanton Morley, Dereham, Norfolk NR20 4NR. Tel: 1362 83767
SAFTA (*Support after Termination for Fetal Abnormality*), 29–30 Soho Square, London W1V 6JB. Tel: 01-439 6124

Postnatal support
Association for Post-Natal Illness, 7 Gowan Avenue, London SW6.
Meet-a-Mum Association (MAMA), 5 Westbury Gardens, Luton, Beds LU2 7DW. Tel: 0582 422253
National Childbirth Trust (as above).

Breast-feeding help and support
Breast-feeding Promotion Group, National Childbirth Trust (as above).
Association of Breast-feeding Mothers, 18 Lucas Court, Winchfield Road, London SE26 5TJ. Tel: 01-778 4769
La Leche League, BM 3424, London WC1V 3XX. Tel: 01-242 1278

Premature babies
Nippers, Sam Segal Perinatal Unit, St Mary's Hospital, Praed Street, London W2. Tel: 01-725 0469

USEFUL ADDRESSES

National Association for the Welfare of Children in Hospital, Argyle House, 29–31 Euston Road, London NW1. Tel: 01-833 2041

Twins
Twins and Multiple Births Association, 292 Valley Road, Lillington, Leamington Spa, Warwickshire CV32 7VE. Tel: 0926 22688

Stillbirth
Stillbirth and Neonatal Death Society, 28 Portland Place, London W1N 3DE. Tel: 01-436-5881
Compassionate Friends, 6 Denmark Street, Bristol B51 5DQ. Tel: 0272 292788

Caesarean section
Caesarean Support Network, 11 Duke Street, Astley, Manchester N29 7BG. Tel: 0942 878076
Caesarean Support Group of Cambridge, 81 Elizabeth Way, Cambridge. Tel: 0223 314211

Private Midwives
Independent Midwives Association, 35 Cleveland Road, London SW13. Tel: 01-278 6783

Pre-eclampsia
Pre-eclamptic Toxaemia Society, 8 Southend Road, Hockley, Essex SS5 4QQ. Tel: 0702 205088

Other useful organizations
Association for Improvements in the Maternity Services, 163 Liverpool Road, London N1. Tel: 01-278 5628 (secretary's address); 21 Iver Lane, Iver, Bucks SL0 9LH. Tel: 0753 652781 (chairperson's address)
Association of Radical Midwives, 8a The Drive, London SW20. Tel: 01-505 2010
Birthright, 27 Sussex Place, Regent's Park, London NW1 4SP. Tel: 01-723 9296
Bumpsadaisy, 43 The Market, Covent Garden, London WC2E 8HA. Tel: 01-836 1105.
Maternity Alliance, 59–61 Camden High Street, London NW1 7LJ. Tel: 01-388 6337
Vegetarian Society, 53 Marloes Road, London W8 6LA. Tel: 01-937 7739
Vegan Society, 33 George Street, Oxford OX1 2AY. Tel: 0865 722166

Useful Reading

Janet Balaskas, *Active Birth*, Unwin Paperbacks.
Janet Balaskas, *The Active Birth Partners' Handbook*, Sidgwick and Jackson.
Janet Balaskas and Yehudi Gordon, *Encyclopaedia of Pregnancy and Childbirth*, Macdonald/Orbis.
Complete Mothercare Manual, from Mothercare by Post, PO Box 145, Watford, Herts (and branches of Mothercare).
Judy Dunn, *Sisters and Brothers*, Fontana.
Barbara Glover and Christine Hodson, *You and Your Premature Baby*, Sheldon Press.
David Harvey (ed.) *A New Life, Pregnancy, Birth and Your Child's First Year*, Hamlyn.
Sheila Kitzinger, *Pregnancy and Childbirth*, Penguin.
Sheila Kitzinger, *Freedom and Choice in Childbirth*, Penguin.
Catharine Lewis, *Good Food Before Birth*, Unwin Paperbacks.
National Childbirth Trust, *The Baby Annual* (available from the NCT address on page 203).
Maire Messenger, *The Breastfeeding Book*, Century.
Barbara Pickard, *Eating Well for a Healthy Pregnancy*, Sheldon Press.
Johanna Roeber, *Shared Parenthood, A Handbook for Fathers*, Century.
Miriam Stoppard, *The Baby Care Book, A Practical Guide to the First Three Years*, Dorling Kindersley.
Marianne Velmans and Sarah Litvinoff, *Working Mother, A Practical Handbook*, Corgi.
Vivienne Welburn, *Postnatal Depression*, Fontana.

Cassettes and Videotapes
Understanding Pregnancy and Birth. A study pack which includes a video of birth produced by the Open University. Write to The Learning Materials Service Office, The Open University, PO Box 188, Milton Keynes MK7 6DH
Shape up for Motherhood. Cassette tape of antenatal and postnatal exercises by Janet Balaskas. Available from the Active Birth Movement (address on page 203).
Active Birth. Video of 2 active births in London. For hire or sale from the Active Birth Movement (address on page 203).

INDEX

Abruptio placenta, 90, 148
Acceleration of labour, 41
Active birth, 40
  classes, 77
Alcohol, 65
Allergies, 64
Alpha-feto protein test, 23, 32
Amenity beds, 38
Amniocentesis, 29–30
Amnioscopy, 32
Antenatal
  care, 17–25
  hospital personnel, 21–3
  tests, 17–18, 19–20, 23–5, 26–33, 142
  see also Classes
Antepartum haemorrhage, 89
Anterior lip, 134
Apgar score, 159
Artificial rupture of membranes, 42, 143
Assertiveness, 47, 49

Baby
  appearance of, 159–60
  blues, 177–8, 188
  crying, 182
  effect on marriage, 183–4
  first days, 157–60
  reflexes, 161–2
  size of, 119
  tests, 161, 162
Backache, 81–2
  in labour, 133, 136
Balaskas, Janet, 40
Benefits, 105–10
Birth Centre classes, 77
Birth options, 39–45
Birth plan, 45–6
Birthing beds, 40
Bleeding
  after delivery, 175
  in late pregnancy, 89
Blood pressure, 23–4
  see also Pre-eclampsia
Blood tests, 19, 23
Bottle-feeding, 51–3, 55, 96, 170–73
Bras, 54, 79–80
Braxton-Hicks contractions, 10, 11, 90, 102, 120
Breaking waters
  artificial, 42, 143
  spontaneous, 120, 126
Breast
  changes, 8, 9, 13, 173–4
  examination, 25
Breast-feeding, 50–51, 53–4, 163–70
  equipment, 95, 96–8
Breathing
  exercises, 132–3
  in a new baby, 157–8
Breathlessness, 82
Breech birth, 113, 115, 150–52

Caesarean, 42, 147–50
  for breech birth, 151–2
Cardiotocograph, 128
Changes in pregnancy, 8–11
Children, older, 100–101
Choice of birthplace, 34–9
Chorion villus sampling, 30–31
Classes, antenatal, 9, 11, 99, 138
  NHS, 74–5
  private, 76–7
Clothing
  for baby, 94, 96
  for you, 77–80
Colostrum, 10
Companion in labour, 43, 127, 131–2, 138–40
Conception, 3
Confinement to bed, 43
Constipation, 82, 176

INDEX

Consultant
  care, 21
  choice of, 39
  unit, 35
Contraception, 186–8
Contractions, 122–6
Co-operation card, 20, 26–7
Cots, 96
Counselling, 184
Cramp, 82–3
Cravings, 59
Cystitis, 83

Delivery room/labour room transfer, 44
Depression, 177–8, 179, 188–90
Diagnosis of pregnancy, 12–14
Diet, 55–64
Doctors
  hierarchies of, 22–3
  see also Consultants, General practitioners
Domino birth scheme, 35, 127
Doppler scan, 7, 28, 91
Down's syndrome, 31, 33
Drips, 42, 123, 143
Drugs, 42, 66, 134–5

Eating
  during pregnancy, 55–64
  in labour, 132
Eclampsia, 91
Embryo, growth of, 3–4
Emergency birth, 137
Emotions, 98–101
Employment rights and benefits, 102–10
Enema, 43, 127
Engagement of baby's head, 117
Entonox, 136
Epidural, 91, 123, 131, 135–6
  for caesarian, 149
Episiotomy, 42, 115, 145–6, 175
Equipment
  for baby, 95, 96–8
  for bottle-feeding, 96
  for breast-feeding, 95
Exercise
  in pregnancy, 67–73
  postnatal, 174, 176, 177
Expressing breast milk, 163, 168–9
Expected date of delivery, 15, 16, 140

Fathers, 18, 99–100, 138–40, 170
Fatigue, 13–14, 85, 178
Feelings, 98–101, 157, 177
Fetal growth, 3–5
Fetal heart monitoring, 25, 26, 32, 41–2
Fetoscopy, 31
Food; *see* Diet
Forceps delivery, 146–7

Gas and air, 136
General practitioners, 14
  and home births, 38
  birth unit, 35
Gestational diabetes, 92
Guthrie test, 162

Haemorrhoids, 83
Hair, 81
Hands, tingling or numb, 85
Health visitor, 180–81
Heartburn, 9, 83
HCG hormone, 3, 12, 84
High-tech birth, 41
Hip dislocation, congenital, 161
Home birth, 34–5, 36–7, 38, 48–9
Hospital
  birth, 34
  booking visit, 18–20
  journey to, 118
  packing for, 93–4
  personnel, 21–3
  private, 38
  procedures, 126–30
  questions for, 45
  when to go to, 125–6
Husbands; *see* Fathers

ICBU (intensive care baby unit), 152
Implantation, 3
Induction, 41, 90, 142–4
Insomnia, 84
Internal examination, 20, 24
Intervention, chain of, 39–40
Iron, 58–9, 82

INDEX

Jaundice, 153

Ketones, 127
Kick chart, 31, 33

Labour, 119–38
 false, 123
 length of, 123–5
 long, 144–5
 pain in, 130–38
 positions for, 117–19
 second stage, 44
 start of, 5, 7, 120
 wards, 127
Leboyer, Frederick, 41, 77
Let-down reflex, 165
Lithotomies, 151
Lochia, 175

Massage, 133
Maternity
 allowance, 110
 leave, 105–6
 pay, 106–7
Meconium test, 162
Midwife
 care, 21
 hierarchies, 22
 postnatal, 180
 private, 35–7
 team, 17
Miscarriage, 86–8
Monitoring, 41–2, 127, 128–30

National Childbirth Trust, 34, 76, 87
Natural birth, 39–40
Nausea and vomiting, 8, 13, 84
Nosebleeds, 85
Nursery, 98

Odent, Michel, 40, 77
Oestriol tests, 31

Packing for hospital, 93–4
Pain, 130–31
 relief, 42, 131–8
Parenthood, 190–93

Partners; *see* Companion in labour,
  Fathers
Partogram, 130
Pelvic floor, 176
Periods, missed, 12–13
Pethidine, 134–5
Piles, 83
Placenta, 7–8, 27
 abruptio, 90, 148
 praevia, 27, 36, 90, 148
Positions
 for delivery, 44
 for labour, 117–18
Postnatal checkup, 185–6
Prams, 97
Precipitate labour, 137
Pre-eclampsia, 7, 18, 24, 25, 90–92, 142
Pregnancy testing, 12, 15
Premature babies, 152–4
Presentation, 44, 113–15
Prostaglandins, 143, 144
Pushchairs, 97

Questions for hospitals, 45

Reflexes in new baby, 161–2
Relaxation, 74
Rhesus factor, 88–9
Rights at work, 105–7
Routine, 181–2
Rubella, 23, 185

SAFTA, 30, 203
Scans; *see* Doppler, Ultrasound
SCBU (special care baby unit), 152
Sex, 101–2, 144, 184
Shared care, 21
Shaving, 43, 127, 148
Signs of pregnancy, 12–14
Skin, appearance of, 80
Smoking, 65–6
Social Fund Maternity Payment, 110
Sonicaid, 128
Stillbirth, 141
Stress tests, 32, 142–3
Sugar in the urine, 92
Sweating, 9, 77

INDEX

Teeth and gums, 81
Telemetry, 128
TENS (transcutaneous electrical nerve stimulation), 133–4, 150
Tests
  antenatal, 17–18, 19–20, 23–5, 26–33, 142
  in labour, 127
  of new baby, 161, 162
Thrush, 85
Tiredness, 85, 178
  see also Fatigue
Transverse presentation, 115
Travel, 66–7
Twins, 115–17

Ultrasound scan, 4, 9, 13, 20, 25, 26–8, 116
Umbilical cord, 41
Urinary frequency, 14

Urine
  retention, 175
  testing, 18, 24

Vaginal examination, 20, 24
Varicose veins, 86
VDUs, 103
Vegan diet, 64
Vegetarian diet, 64
Ventouse delivery, 146–7
Vernix, 4–5
Visitors, 180
Vitamins and minerals, 60–63, 66

Water birth, 41
Waters breaking; *see* Breaking waters
Weight gain and loss, 10, 24, 59–60
Work, 102–6
Worries, 99

Mother & Baby
MAGAZINE

your pregnancy and childcare expert

With a baby on the way, it is important to keep track of the latest developments on all aspects of motherhood, from conception through to the early years with your new baby.

Mother & Baby magazine is Britain's best monthly guide, packed with exclusive reports and lively features for you and your growing family.

Regular sections on pregnancy and birth, your baby and toddler, family relationships and health and medicine offer factual information and expert advice which will continue to support you throughout the coming months and years ... Plus a special colour section on the lighter side of motherhood, with fashion tips for you and your child, things to make and do, and lots of free gifts and special offers in every issue.

So make sure you don't miss a single issue of **Mother & Baby**. Have the next 12 issues delivered straight to your door, postage free, for only £12.00 – plus a full money-back guarantee if you decide to cancel at any time!

Simply call our *Subscription Hotline* direct on 0235 865656 with details of your Access or Visa card, and we'll take care of the rest. Or, if you prefer, complete the coupon below and post the whole page to:

Mother & Baby, FREEPOST, PO Box 35, Abingdon, Oxon OX14 3BR.

Yes, please send me the next 12 issues of **Mother & Baby** magazine, for only £12.00, postage free. I understand I can cancel at any time and receive a full refund.

Name
Address

Postcode   Tel. no.
                  A8490

I enclose cheque/PO for £
made payable to **Mother & Baby**

Please debit £
to my Access/Visa card, no.

Signature

Expiry date